Free Video

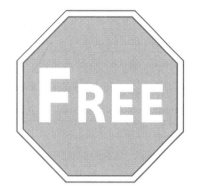

Free Video

Essential Test Tips Video from Trivium Test Prep

Dear Customer,

Thank you for purchasing from Trivium Test Prep! We're honored to help you prepare for your PSB APNE exam.

To show our appreciation, we're offering a **FREE *PSB APNE Essential Test Tips* Video by Trivium Test Prep.*** Our video includes 35 test preparation strategies that will make you successful on the PSB APNE. All we ask is that you email us your feedback and describe your experience with our product. Amazing, awful, or just so-so: we want to hear what you have to say!

To receive your **FREE *PSB APNE Essential Test Tips* Video**, please email us at 5star@ triviumtestprep.com. Include "Free 5 Star" in the subject line and the following information in your email:

1. The title of the product you purchased.
2. Your rating from 1 – 5 (with 5 being the best).
3. Your feedback about the product, including how our materials helped you meet your goals and ways in which we can improve our products.
4. Your full name and shipping address so we can send your **FREE *PSB APNE Essential Test Tips* Video.**

If you have any questions or concerns please feel free to contact us directly at 5star@ triviumtestprep.com.

Thank you!

– Trivium Test Prep Team

*To get access to the free video please email us at 5star@triviumtestprep.com, and please follow the instructions above.

PSB PRACTICAL NURSING EXAM STUDY GUIDE 2019–2020

Nursing Exam Prep Book and Practice Test Questions for the PSB Aptitude for Practical Nursing Examination

TABLE OF CONTENTS

Online Resources i

Introduction iii

ONE: Verbal Skills 1
WORD STRUCTURE........................ 1
PREFIXES.................................3
SUFFIXES.................................4
MEDICAL TERMINOLOGY 5
TEST YOUR KNOWLEDGE....................11

TWO: Arithmetic....................13
MATHEMATICAL OPERATIONS 13
OPERATIONS WITH POSITIVE AND NEGATIVE NUMBERS 14
FRACTIONS.............................15
DECIMALS 17
CONVERTING FRACTIONS AND DECIMALS 19
RATIOS 19
PROPORTIONS...........................20
PERCENTS 21
ESTIMATION AND ROUNDING 21
STATISTICS 22
UNITS 23
TEST YOUR KNOWLEDGE....................27

THREE: Nonverbal Subtest 31
WHAT IS AN ANALOGY?....................31
NONVERBAL ANALOGIES....................32
TEST YOUR KNOWLEDGE....................35

FOUR: Spelling 37
SPELLING RULE ONE: PLURALS 37
SPELLING RULE TWO: CONJUGATING VERBS 38
SPELLING RULE THREE: I BEFORE E........39
SPELLING RULE FOUR: SUFFIXES..............39
COMMONLY MISSPELLED WORDS.............39
TEST YOUR KNOWLEDGE....................43

FIVE: Life Science 45
BIOLOGICAL MOLECULES.....................45
NUCLEIC ACIDS 47
STRUCTURE AND FUNCTION OF CELLS 48
CELLULAR RESPIRATION 50
PHOTOSYNTHESIS 51
CELL DIVISION 52
GENETICS..............................54
EVOLUTION 55
ECOLOGY 57
HUMAN ANATOMY AND PHYSIOLOGY.......59
TEST YOUR KNOWLEDGE....................67

SIX: Physical Science 73
THE STRUCTURE OF THE ATOM 73
THE PERIODIC TABLE OF THE ELEMENTS 76
CHEMICAL BONDS 77
PROPERTIES OF MATTER 78
STATES OF MATTER......................79
CHEMICAL REACTIONS....................80

Mixtures 82

Acids and Bases......................83

Motion 85

Forces 86

Work 87

Energy 88

Waves 90

Electricity and Magnetism 92

Test Your Knowledge 95

SEVEN: Earth and
Space Science 103

Astronomy 103

Geology..................................... 104

Hydrology 106

Meteorology............................... 109

Test Your Knowledge.......................... 111

EIGHT: Judgment
and Comprehension................. 115

Scope of Practice for the
Practical Nurse 115

Therapeutic Communication 116

Reporting to the Supervisor 117

Privacy 117

Test Your Knowledge...................... 119

NINE: Vocational
Adjustment Index......................121

TEN: Practice Test 123

Answer Key 147

ONLINE RESOURCES

To help you fully prepare for your Aptitude for Practical Nursing Examination (APNE), Ascencia includes online resources with the purchase of this study guide.

PRACTICE TEST

In addition to the practice test included in this book, we also offer an online exam. Since many exams today are computer based, getting to practice your test-taking skills on the computer is a great way to prepare.

FLASH CARDS

A convenient supplement to this study guide, Ascencia's flash cards enable you to review important terms easily on your computer or smartphone.

CHEAT SHEETS

Review the core skills you need to master the exam with easy-to-read Cheat Sheets.

FROM STRESS TO SUCCESS

Watch "From Stress to Success," a brief but insightful YouTube video that offers the tips, tricks, and secrets experts use to score higher on the exam.

REVIEWS

Leave a review, send us helpful feedback, or sign up for Ascencia promotions—including free books!

Access these materials at:

http://ascenciatestprep.om/psb-apne-online-resources

INTRODUCTION

The Aptitude for Practical Nursing Examination (APNE) was developed by the Psychological Services Bureau (PSB) for use by practical and vocational nursing programs during the application process. The exam evaluates candidates' relevant knowledge and skills so that they can be accurately placed in nursing education programs.

What's on the APNE?

The APNE is a multiple-choice test. It includes concepts covered in eighth grade-level English, math, and science classes; it will also test your ability to identify relationships between shapes. It also includes a short vocational test to measure your personal suitability to work in health care. Finally, the APNE includes a section designed to gauge your understanding of professional behavior for practical and vocational nurses.

Test	Concepts	Number of Questions	Time
Part I: Academic Aptitude	**Verbal Subtest**: identifying related vocabulary words	75	40 minutes
	Arithmetic Subtest: performing arithmetic calculations		
	Nonverbal Subtest: identifying patterns in shapes		
Part II: Spelling Test	identifying misspelled words	45	15 minutes
Part III: Information in the Natural Sciences	answering questions about biology, chemistry, physics, and health	60	25 minutes
Part IV: Judgment and Comprehension in Practical Nursing Situations	using personal judgment to answer questions about workplace scenarios	40	25 minutes

Test	Concepts	Number of Questions	Time
Part V: Vocational Adjustment Index	choosing to agree or disagree with statements about your personality and workplace behaviors	90	15 minutes
Total		**310 questions**	**2 hours**

Note: Number of questions and time may vary.

How is the APNE Administered?

The APNE is administered by individual health care education programs. Most programs will require you to take the test at a specified testing location, usually on their campus. You should check with the program to which you are applying to find testing dates and locations. If you want to report your APNE score to a school at which you did not test, you will need to contact the school's admissions office.

Before you take the APNE, carefully check the policies and procedures for your particular test site. Fees and payment methods will vary by school. In addition, most schools will have specific requirements for what you will need to bring (e.g., identification, pencils) and what not to bring (e.g., calculators, cell phones).

The PSB allows you to re-take the APNE. However, each school will have its own policy about which scores they will accept. Keep in mind that schools may require you to take the APNE the same year that you are applying.

How is the APNE Scored?

You will receive a raw score and a percentile rank for each of the five tests and three subtests. The raw score will simply show how many questions you answered correctly. The percentile rank will show how you scored compared to other candidates. For example, if you are in the seventy-fifth percentile for the Reading Comprehension test, that means you scored higher than 75 percent of all test takers. If you test at the health care education program to which you are applying, they will be sent a copy of your results.

There is no set "passing" score for the APNE. Each program will have its own guidelines for how it interprets your scores during the application review process. Contact your school's admissions office if you would like to learn more about how they use APNE score reports.

Ascencia Test Prep

With health care fields such as nursing, pharmacy, emergency care, and physical therapy becoming the fastest-growing industries in the United States, individuals looking to enter the health care industry or rise in their field need high-quality, reliable resources. Ascencia Test Prep's study guides and test preparation materials are developed by credentialed industry professionals with years of experience in their respective fields. Ascencia recognizes that health care professionals nurture bodies and spirits, and save lives. Ascencia Test Prep's mission is to help health care workers grow.

ONE: VERBAL SKILLS

The thirty verbal questions on the Academic Aptitude test will gauge your knowledge of common vocabulary words. You will see a list of five words labeled *a* through *e*, and your job is to find the word that doesn't fit with the others.

Verbal Question Format

Which word is most different in meaning from the other words?

1.   a. kind b. gracious c. friendly d. vicious e. considerate

Fortunately, to answer these questions, you don't have to know the exact definition of all the words. Usually you'll just need to pick out the word that doesn't match in tone. Having a large vocabulary will obviously help with these questions, but you can also use root words and affixes to determine the meaning of unfamiliar words.

Word Structure

An unfamiliar word itself can provide clues about its meaning. Most words consist of discrete pieces that determine their meaning; these pieces include word roots, prefixes, and suffixes.

Word roots are the bases from which many words take their form and meaning. The most common word roots are Greek and Latin, and a broad knowledge of these roots can make it much easier to determine the meaning of words.

Table 1.1. Common Word Roots

Root	Meaning	Examples
alter	other	alternate
ambi	both	ambidextrous
ami, amic	love	amiable
amphi	both ends, all sides	amphibian

Table 1.1. Common Word Roots (continued)

Root	Meaning	Examples
aqua	water	aqueduct
aud	to hear	audience
auto	self	autobiography
bell	war	belligerent
bene	good	benevolent
bio	life	biology
ced	yield, go	secede
chron	time	chronological
circum	around	circumference
contra, counter	against	contradict
crypt	hidden	cryptic
curr, curs, cours	to run	precursory
dict	to say	dictator
dyna	power	dynamic
dys	bad, hard, unlucky	dysfunctional
equ	equal, even	equanimity
fort	strength	fortitude
fract	to break	fracture
grad, gress	step	progression
graph	writing	graphic
hetero	different	heterogeneous
homo	same	homogenous
hypo	below, beneath	hypothermia
ject	throw	projection
logy	study of	biology
luc	light	elucidate
mal	bad	malevolent
meta, met	behind, between	metacognition
mis, miso	hate	misanthrope
morph	form, shape	morphology
mort	death	mortal
multi	many	multiple
path	feeling, disease	apathy

Root	Meaning	Examples
phil	love	philanthropist
port	carry	transportation
pseudo	false	pseudonym
psycho	soul, spirit	psychic
rupt	to break	disruption
sect, sec	to cut	section
sequ, secu	follow	consecutive
soph	wisdom, knowledge	philosophy
tele	far off	telephone
terr	earth	terrestrial
therm	heat	thermal
vent, vene	to come	convene

Prefixes

In addition to understanding the base of a word, it's helpful to know common affixes that change the meaning of words and demonstrate their relationships to other words. **Prefixes** are added to the beginning of words and frequently change their meaning (sometimes even to the opposite meaning).

Table 1.2. Common Prefixes

Prefix	Meaning	Examples
a, an	without, not	anachronism
ab, abs, a	apart, away from	abnormal
ad	toward	adhere
ante	before	anterior
anti	against	antipathy
bi	two	binary
circum	around	circumnavigate
di	two, double	diatomic
dia	across, through	dialectic
dis	not, apart	disenfranchise
ego	I, self	egomaniac
epi	upon, over	epigram, epiphyte
ex	out	extraneous

Table 1.2. Common Prefixes (continued)

Prefix	Meaning	Examples
ideo	idea	ideology
in, im	not	immoral
inter	between	interstellar
locus	place	locality
macro	large	macrophage
micro	small	micron
mono	one, single	monocle
poly	many	polygamy
pre	before	prescient
sym	with	symbiosis
un	not	unsafe

Suffixes

Suffixes are added to the end of words, and like prefixes they modify the meaning of the word root. Suffixes also serve an important grammatical function and can change a part of speech or indicate if a word is plural or related to a plural.

Table 1.3. Common Suffixes		
Suffix	**Meaning**	**Examples**
able, ible	able, capable	visible
age	act of, state of, result of	wreckage
an, ian	native of, relating to	vegetarian
ance, ancy	action, process, state	defiance
ary, ery, ory	relating to, quality, place	aviary
cian	possessing a specific skill or art	physician
cule, ling	very small	sapling
cy	action, function	normalcy
dom	quality, realm	wisdom
ee	one who receives the action	nominee
en	made of, to make	silken
ence, ency	action, state of, quality	urgency
er, or	one who, that which	professor

Suffix	Meaning	Examples
escent	in the process of	adolescent
esis, osis	action, process, condition	neurosis
fic	making, causing	specific
ful	full of	frightful
hood	order, condition, quality	adulthood
ice	condition, state, quality	malice
ile	relating to, suited for, capable of	juvenile
ine	nature of	feminine
ion, sion, tion	act, result, state of	contagion
ish	origin, nature, resembling	impish
ism	system, manner, condition, characteristic	capitalism
ist	one who, that which	artist
ite	nature of, quality of, mineral product	graphite
ity, ty	state of, quality	captivity
ive	causing, making	exhaustive
ment	act of, state of, result	containment
some	like, apt, tending to	gruesome
tude	state of, condition of	aptitude
ure	state of, act, process, rank	rupture
y	inclined to, tend to	faulty

Medical Terminology

Below is a list of common medical terms that may appear on the verbal or spelling sections of the test.

abate: become less in amount or intensity

abduction: the movement of a limb away from the body's midline

abbreviate: to shorten or abridge

abrasion: an area of the skin damaged by scraping or wearing away

absorb: to take in

abstain: refrain; choose to avoid or not participate

access: means of approach or admission

accountable: liable or responsible

acoustic: related to sound or hearing

acuity: sharpness of vision or hearing; mental quickness

adhere: hold closely to an idea or course; be devoted

adverse: harmful to one's interests; unfortunate

amalgam: a mixture or blend

ambulatory: able to walk

analgesic: a drug that relieves pain

anomaly: something unusual

aphasia: impairment in ability to speak, write, and understand others

apnea: temporary cessation of breathing

aseptic: free from bacteria and other pathogens

attenuate: to weaken

audible: loud enough to be heard

benevolent: showing sympathy, understanding, and generosity

benign: not harmful; not malignant

bias: an unfair preference or dislike

bilateral: having two sides

bradycardia: slow heart rate

bradypnea: slow respiration rate

cannula: a thin tube inserted into the body to collect or drain fluid

cardiac: pertaining to the heart

cease: stop doing an action, discontinue

cephalic: relating to the head

chronic: persistent or recurring over a long time period

co-morbidity: two disorders that occur at the same time

cohort: a group of people who are treated as a group

collaborate: work together on a common project

collateral: adjoining or accompanying

compassion: awareness and sympathy for the experiences and suffering of others

complication: something intricate, involved, or aggravating

comply: acquiesce to another's wish, command, etc.

compression: pressing together

compromise: an accommodation in which both sides make concessions

concave: with an outline or surface curved inward

concise: brief and compact

conditional: dependent on something else being done

consistency: state of being congruous; conforming to regular patterns, habits, principles, etc.

constrict: cause to shrink, cramp, crush

contingent: depending on something not certain; conditional

contraindication: discouragement of the use of a treatment

copious: abundant and plentiful

culture: the growth of microorganisms in an artificial environment

cyanosis: blueish skin

defecate: have a bowel movement

deleterious: harmful or deadly to living things

depress: weaken; sadden

depth: deepness; distance measured downward, inward, or backward

dermal: relating to skin

deter: to prevent or discourage

deteriorating: growing worse; reducing in worth; impairing

diagnosis: analysis of a present condition

dilate: expand; make larger

diligent: persistent and hardworking

dilute: weaken by a mixture of water or other liquid; reduce in strength

discrete: separate; discontinuous

dysphagia: difficulty swallowing

dyspnea: difficulty breathing

dysuria: difficult or painful urination

ecchymosis: bruising

edema: swelling caused by excess fluid

elevate: raise; lift up

empathy: understanding of another's feelings

endogenous: something produced within the body

enervating: causing debilitation or weakness

enhance: to improve; to increase clarity

enteral: relating to the small intestine

ephemeral: lasting only for a short period of time

epistaxis: bleeding from the nose

erythema: redness of the skin

exacerbate: make more bitter, angry, or violent; irritate or aggravate

excess: the state of being more or too much; a surplus or remainder

exogenous: something produced outside the body

expand: increase in extent, bulk, or amount; spread or stretch out; unfold

exposure: the state of being exposed or open to external environments

extenuating: diminish the seriousness of something

external: located outside of something and/ or apart from something

fatal: causing death or ruin

fatigue: weariness from physical or mental exertion

febrile: related to fever

flaccid: soft; flabby

flushed: suffused with color; washed out with a copious flow of water

focal: centered in one area

gaping: to be open; to have a break in continuity

gastric: relating to the stomach

hematologic: dealing with the blood

hepatic: relating to the living

hydration: the act of meeting body fluid demands

hygiene: the science that deals with the preservation of health

hypertension: high blood pressure

hypotension: low blood pressure

imminent: very likely to happen

impaired: made worse, damaged, or weakened

incidence: frequency or range of occurrence; extent of effects

incompatible: unable to be or work together

infection: tainted with germs or disease

inflamed: condition in which the body is inflicted with heat, swelling, and redness

ingest: take into the body for digestion

initiate: set going; begin; originate

innocuous: harmless

intact: remaining uninjured, unimpaired, whole, or complete

internal: situated within something; enclosed; inside

intuitive: to know by instinct alone

invasive: being intrusive or encroaching upon

ischemia: restricted blood flow to tissue

jaundice: yellowing of the skin or sclera

jerk: a quick, sudden movement

labile: unstable

laceration: a rough tear; an affliction

languid: tired and slow

latent: hidden; dormant; undeveloped

lethargic: not wanting to move; sluggish

longevity: having a long life

malady: a disease or disorder

malaise: a general feeling of illness or discomfort

malignant: harmful

manifestation: a demonstration or display

musculoskeletal: pertaining to muscles and the skeleton

neurologic: dealing with the nervous system

neurovascular: pertaining to the nervous system and blood vessels

nexus: a connection or series of connections

novice: a beginner; inexperienced

nutrient: something affording nutrition

obverse: the opposite

occluded: shut in or out; closed; absorbed

occult: hidden

oral: spoken, not written; pertaining to the mouth

ossify: to harden

overt: plain to the view; open

palliate: to lessen symptoms without treating the underlying cause

pallor: pale appearance

paroxysmal: having to do with a spasm or violent outburst

pathogenic: causing disease

pathology: the science of the nature and origin of disease

posterior: located in the back or rear

potent: wielding power; strong; effective

pragmatic: concerned with practical matters and results

precaution: an act done in advance to ensure safety or benefit; prudent foresight

predispose: give a tendency or inclination to; dispose in advance

preexisting: already in place; already occurring

primary: first; earliest; most important

priority: right of precedence; order of importance

prognosis: a forecast

prudent: careful and sensible; using good judgment

rationale: rational basis for something; justification

recur: appear again; return

renal: pertaining to the kidneys

regress: to return to a former state

resect: to remove or cut out

resilient: quick to recover

respiration: breathing

restrict: attach limitations to; restrain

retain: hold or keep in possession, use, or practice

shunt: a tube that diverts the path of a fluid in the body

soporific: a drug that induces sleep

status: relative standing; position; condition

pallor: pale appearance

sublingual: beneath the tongue

subtle: understated, not obvious

succumb: to stop resisting

superficial: shallow in character and attitude; only concerned with things on the surface

superfluous: more than is needed, desired, or necessary

supplement: an addition to something substantially completed; to add to

suppress: restrain; abolish; repress

symmetric: similar proportion in the size or shape of something

symptom: a sign or indication of a problem or disease

syncope: temporary loss of consciousness

syndrome: a set of symptoms that characterize a certain disease or condition

systemic: affecting the whole body

tachycardia: fast heart rate

tachypnea: fast respiratory rate

therapeutic: pertaining to the curing of disease; having remedial effect

transdermal: passing through the skin

transient: lasting for only a short time or duration

transmission: the act or result of sending something along or onward to a recipient or destination

trauma: a bodily injury or mental shock

triage: the act of sorting or categorizing conditions and diseases in preparation for treatment

unilateral: relating to only one side

vascular: pertaining to bodily ducts that convey fluid

vertigo: sensation of dizziness and loss of balance

virus: an agent of infection

vital: pertaining to life; alive; essential to existence or well-being

void: empty; evacuate

volume: the amount of space occupied by a substance

Test Your Knowledge

Which word is most different in meaning from the other words?

1.	a. malice	b. hatred	c. animosity	d. hostility	e. sympathy
2.	a. condense	b. augment	c. boost	d. enlarge	e. expand
3.	a. serene	b. peaceful	c. agitated	d. tranquil	e. quiet
4.	a. bellow	b. shout	c. howl	d. whimper	e. shriek
5.	a. cease	b. persist	c. continue	d. remain	e. endure
6.	a. flourish	b. prosper	c. thrive	d. shrivel	e. multiply
7.	a. obscured	b. apparent	c. evident	d. clear	e. obvious
8.	a. sparse	b. plentiful	c. scant	d. meager	e. thin
9.	a. concur	b. agree	c. oppose	d. approve	e. unite
10.	a. deadly	b. benign	c. lethal	d. fatal	e. harmful

1. e.

Sympathy means "feeling pity or understanding for somebody"; the other four words describe negative emotions.

2. a.

Condense means to "make smaller or more compact," and the other four words mean to make larger.

3. c.

Agitated means disturbed or upset, and the other four words describe the feeling of being calm.

4. d.

Whimper means to "make a low whining sound," and the other four words describe making loud sounds.

5. a.

Cease means stop, and the other four words mean to keep going.

6. d.

Shrivel means shrink, and the other four words mean to become larger or better.

7. a.

Obscured means "to be hidden," and the other four words describe things that can be easily seen.

8. b.

Plentiful means "present in large amounts," and the other four words describe a small supply.

9. c.

Oppose means "go against," and the other four words mean to agree or go along with.

10. b.

Benign means "harmless," and the other four words describe something dangerous.

TWO: ARITHMETIC

The twenty arithmetic questions will require you to read word problems and perform calculations to find the answer. You will not be able to use a calculator.

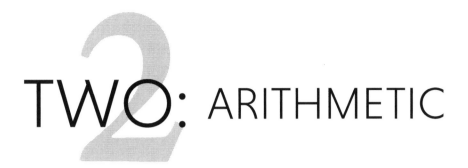

Arithmetic Question Format

1. A nurse has 25 patients to see in a day. If she has seen 13 patients, how many patients still need to be seen?

a. 7 b. 8 c. 12 d. 13 e. 38

Mathematical Operations

The four basic arithmetic operations are addition, subtraction, multiplication, and division.

- ✦ **Add** to combine two quantities (6 + 5 = 11).
- ✦ **Subtract** to find the difference of two quantities (10 − 3 = 7).
- ✦ **Multiply** to add a quantity multiple times (4 × 3 = 12).
- ✦ **Divide** to find out how many times one quantity goes into another (10 ÷ 2 = 5).

On the exam, operations questions will often be word problems. These problems will contain **clue words** that help you determine which operation to use.

Table 2.1. Operations Word Problems

Operation	Clue Words	Example
Addition	sum, together, (in) total, all, in addition, increased, give	Leslie has 3 pencils. If her teacher **gives** her 2 pencils, how many does she now have **in total**? 3 + 2 = 5 pencils
Subtraction	minus, less than, take away, decreased, difference, How many left?, How many more/less?	Sean has 12 cookies. His sister **takes** 2 cookies. **How many** cookies does Sean have **left**? 12 − 2 = 10 cookies

Table 2.1. Operations Word Problems (continued)

Operation	Clue Words	Example
Multiplication	product, times, of, each/every, groups of, twice	A hospital department has 10 patient rooms. If **each** room holds 2 patients, how many patients can stay in the department? 10 × 2 = 20 patients
Division	divided, per, each/every, distributed, average, How many for each?, How many groups?	A teacher has 150 stickers to **distribute** to her class of 25 students. If each student gets the same number of stickers, **how many** stickers will **each** student get? 150 ÷ 25 = 6 stickers

PRACTICE QUESTIONS

1. A case of powder-free nitrile gloves contains 10 boxes. Each box contains 150 gloves. How many gloves are in the case?

Answer:
Multiply the number of boxes by the number of gloves in each box to find the total number of gloves.
10 × 150 = **1500 gloves**

2. A taxi company charges $5 for the first mile traveled, then $1 for each additional mile. What is the cost of a 10-mile taxi ride?

Answer:
The first mile will cost $5, and the additional 9 miles will cost $1 each.
cost = $5 + (9)($1) = **$14**

Operations with Positive and Negative Numbers

Positive numbers are greater than zero, and **negative numbers** are less than zero. Use the rules in Table 2.2 to determine the sign of the answer when performing operations with positive and negative numbers.

 Helpful Hint: Subtracting a negative number is the same as adding a positive number: 5 − (−10) = 5 + (+10) = 5 + 10 = 15

Table 2.2. Operations with Positive and Negative Numbers

Addition and Subtraction	Multiplication and Division
positive + positive = positive 4 + 5 = 9	positive × positive = positive 5 × 3 = 15
negative + negative = negative −4 + −5 = −9 → −4 − 5 = −9	negative × negative = positive −6 × −5 = 30
negative + positive = sign of the larger number −15 + 9 = −6	negative × positive = negative −5 × 4 = −20

A **number line** shows numbers increasing from left to right (usually with zero in the middle). When adding positive and negative numbers, a number line can be used to find the sign of the answer. When adding a positive number, count to the right; when adding a negative number, count to the left. Note that adding a negative value is the same as subtracting.

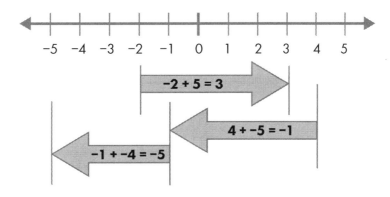

Figure 2.1. Adding Positive and Negative Numbers

PRACTICE QUESTION

3.   The wind chill on a cold day in January was −3°F. When the sun went down, the temperature fell 5 degrees. What was the temperature after the sun went down?

Answer:

Because the temperature went down, add a negative number.

−3 + −5 = **−8°F**

Fractions

A **fraction** represents parts of a whole. The top number of a fraction, called the **numerator**, indicates how many equal-sized parts are present. The bottom number of a fraction, called the **denominator**, indicates how many equal-sized parts make a whole.

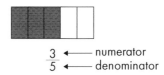

Figure 2.2. Parts of Fractions

Fractions have several forms:

✦ **proper fraction**: the numerator is less than the denominator

✦ **improper fraction**: the numerator is greater than or equal to the denominator

✦ **mixed number**: the combination of a whole number and a fraction

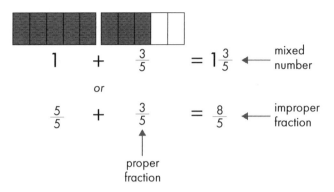

Figure 2.3. Types of Fractions

Improper fractions can be converted to mixed numbers by dividing. In fact, the fraction bar is also a division symbol.

$$\frac{14}{3} = 14 \div 3 = 4 \text{ (with 2 left over)}$$

$$\frac{14}{3} = 4\frac{2}{3}$$

To convert a mixed number to a fraction, multiply the whole number by the denominator of the fraction, and add the numerator. The result becomes the numerator of the improper fraction; the denominator remains the same.

$$5\frac{2}{3} = \frac{(5 \times 3) + 2}{3} = \frac{17}{3}$$

To **multiply fractions**, multiply numerators and multiply denominators. Reduce the product to lowest terms. To **divide fractions**, multiply the dividend (the first fraction) by the reciprocal of the divisor (the fraction that follows the division symbol).

When multiplying and dividing mixed numbers, the mixed numbers must be converted to improper fractions.

 Helpful Hint: The reciprocal of a fraction is just the fraction with the top and bottom numbers switched.

Adding or subtracting fractions requires a common denominator. To find a **common denominator**, multiply the denominators of the fractions. Then, to add the fractions, add the numerators and keep the denominator the same.

PRACTICE QUESTIONS

4. $7\frac{1}{2} \times 1\frac{5}{6} =$

Answer:

Convert the mixed numbers to improper fractions.

$$7\frac{1}{2} = \frac{7 \times 2 + 1}{2} = \frac{15}{2}$$

$$1\frac{5}{6} = \frac{1 \times 6 + 5}{6} = \frac{11}{6}$$

Multiply the numerators, multiply the denominators, and reduce.

$$\frac{15}{2} \times \frac{11}{6} = \frac{165}{12} = \frac{165 \div 3}{12 \div 3} = \mathbf{\frac{55}{4}}$$

5.   Ari and Teagan each ordered a pizza. Ari has $\frac{1}{4}$ of his pizza left, and Teagan has $\frac{1}{3}$ of her pizza left. How much total pizza do they now have?

Answer:

The common denominator is $4 \times 3 = 12$.

Convert each fraction to the common denominator.

$$\frac{1}{4}\left(\frac{3}{3}\right) = \frac{3}{12}$$

$$\frac{1}{3}\left(\frac{4}{4}\right) = \frac{4}{12}$$

Add the numerators and keep the denominator the same.

$$\frac{3}{12} + \frac{4}{12} = \frac{7}{12}$$

Together, they have $\mathbf{\frac{7}{12}}$ **of a pizza**.

Decimals

In the base-10 system, each digit (the numeric symbols 0 – 9) in a number is worth ten times as much as the number to the right of it. For example, in the number 321 each digit has a different value based on its location: 321 = 300 + 20 + 1. The value of each place is called **place value**.

Table 2.3. Place Value Chart									
1,000,000	100,000	10,000	1,000	100	10	1		$\frac{1}{10}$	$\frac{1}{100}$
10^6	10^5	10^4	10^3	10^2	10^1	10^0	.	10^{-1}	10^{-2}
millions	hundred thousands	ten thousands	thousands	hundreds	tens	ones	decimal	tenths	hun-dredths

To **add decimal numbers**, line up digits with the same place value. This can be accomplished by writing the numbers vertically and lining up the decimal points. Add zeros as needed so that all the numbers have the same number of decimal places.

To **subtract decimal numbers**, follow the same procedure: write the numbers vertically, lining up the decimal points and adding zeros as necessary.

It is not necessary to line up decimal points to multiply decimal numbers. Simply multiply the numbers, ignoring the decimal point. Then, add together the total number of decimal places in the factors. The product should have the same number of decimal places as this total.

To **divide decimal numbers**, write the problem in long division format. Move the decimal point in the divisor all the way to the right, so that the divisor is a whole number. Move the decimal point in the dividend the same number of places. Position the decimal point in the quotient directly above its new place in the dividend. Then divide, ignoring the decimal point. If necessary, add zeros to the dividend until there is no remainder.

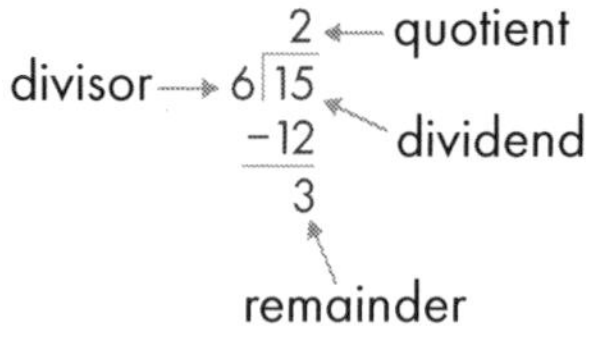

Figure 2.4. Division Terms

PRACTICE QUESTIONS

6. A customer at a restaurant ordered a drink that cost $2.20, a meal that cost $32.54, and a dessert that cost $4. How much was the total bill?

Answer:

Rewrite the numbers vertically, lining up the decimal point.

    2.20
   32.54
 + 4.00
   38.74

The meal cost **$38.74**.

7. 1.324 ÷ 0.05 =

Answer:

The decimal point in the divisor needs to be moved two places to the right, so move it two places to the right in the divisor as well. Then position the decimal point in the quotient.

$$
\begin{array}{r}
\textbf{26.48} \\
005\overline{)132.40} \\
-10 \\
\hline
32 \\
-30 \\
\hline
24 \\
-20 \\
\hline
40 \\
-40 \\
\hline
0
\end{array}
$$

8. A carnival ride rotates 2.15 times per minute. If a rider is on the ride for 3.5 minutes, how many times did the rider rotate?

Answer:

This is a multiplication problem.

$2.15 \times 3.5 =$

First, multiply the factors, ignoring the decimal point.

$215 \times 35 = 7525$

The factors have a total of three decimal places, so the answer is **7.525 rotations**.

Converting Fractions and Decimals

To convert a decimal number to a fraction, write the digits in the numerator and write the place value of the final digit in the denominator. Reduce to lowest terms, if necessary.

To convert a fraction to a decimal, divide the numerator by the denominator.

PRACTICE QUESTIONS

9.　Convert 0.096 to a fraction.

Answer:

The final digit is in the thousandths place, so 0.096 is $\frac{96}{1000}$.

Simplify the fraction by dividing the numerator and the denominator by their greatest common factor.

$$\frac{96 \div 8}{1000 \div 8} = \frac{\mathbf{12}}{\mathbf{125}}$$

10.　Convert $\frac{5}{8}$ to a decimal.

Answer:

$$
\begin{array}{r}
\mathbf{0.625} \\
8\overline{)5.000} \\
-48 \\
\hline
20 \\
-16 \\
\hline
40 \\
-40 \\
\hline
0 \\
\end{array}
$$

Ratios

A **ratio** is a comparison of two quantities. For example, if a class consists of fifteen women and ten men, the ratio of women to men is 15 to 10. This ratio can also be written as 15:10 or $\frac{15}{10}$. Ratios, like fractions, can be reduced by dividing by common factors.

11. A company employs 30 people, 12 of whom are men. What is the ratio of women to men working at the company?

<u>Answer:</u>

Find the number of women working at the company.

30 − 12 = 18 women

Write the ratio as the number of women over the number of men working at the company.

$$\frac{\text{number of women}}{\text{number of men}} = \frac{18}{12}$$

Reduce the ratio.

$$\frac{18 \div 6}{12 \div 6} = \frac{3}{2}$$

The ratio of women to men is $\frac{3}{2}$ or **3:2**.

Proportions

A **proportion** is a statement that two ratios are equal. For example, proportion $\frac{5}{10} = \frac{7}{14}$ is true because both ratios are equal to $\frac{1}{2}$.

The cross product is found by multiplying the top of one fraction by the bottom of the other (*across* the equal sign).

Cross product: $\frac{a}{b} = \frac{c}{d} \rightarrow ad = bc$

Proportions have a useful quality: their cross products are equal.

$$\frac{5}{10} = \frac{7}{14}$$

$$5(14) = 7(10)$$

$$70 = 70$$

The fact that the cross products of proportions are equal can be used to solve proportions in which one of the values is missing. Use x to stand in for the missing variable, then cross multiply and solve.

PRACTICE QUESTION

12. The dosage for a particular medication is proportional to the weight of the patient. If the dosage for a patient weighing 60 kg is 90 mg, what is the dosage for a patient weighing 80 kg?

<u>Answer:</u>

Write a proportion using x for the missing value.

$$\frac{60 \text{ kg}}{90 \text{ mg}} = \frac{80 \text{ kg}}{x \text{ mg}}$$

Cross multiply.

$60(x) = 80(90)$

$60x = 7200$

Divide by 60.

$x = 120$

The proper dosage is **120 mg**.

Percents

A **percent** (or percentage) means *per hundred* and is expressed with the percent symbol, %. For example, 54% means 54 out of every 100. Percents are turned into decimals by moving the decimal point two places to the left, so 54% = 0.54. Percentages can be solved by setting up a proportion:

$$\frac{\text{part}}{\text{whole}} = \frac{\%}{100}$$

PRACTICE QUESTION

13. On one day, a radiology clinic had 80% of patients come in for their scheduled appointments. If they saw 16 patients, how many scheduled appointments did the clinic have that week?

Answer:

Set up a proportion and solve.

$$\frac{\text{part}}{\text{whole}} = \frac{\%}{100}$$

$$\frac{16}{x} = \frac{80}{100}$$

$16(100) = 80(x)$

$x = 20$

There were **20 scheduled appointments** that day.

Estimation and Rounding

Estimation is the process of rounding numbers before performing operations in order to make those operations easier. Estimation can be used when an exact answer is not necessary or to check work.

To round a number, first identify the digit in the specified place. Then look at the digit one place to the right. If that digit is 4 or less, keep the digit in the specified place the same. If that digit is 5 or more, add 1 to the digit in the specified place. All the digits to the right of the specified place become zeros.

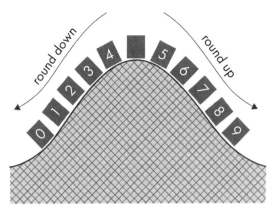

Figure 2.5. Rounding

PRACTICE QUESTION

14. In September, Alicia's electric bill was $49.22, and her water bill was $22.14. Estimate the total of her utilities for September.

Answer:

Solve the problem by rounding the expenses to the nearest $10.

$49.22 rounds up to $50 because the digit in the ones place is 9.

$22.14 rounds down to $20 because the digit in the ones place is 2.

50 + 20 = 70, so Alicia's September utilities are about **$70**.

Statistics

A **measure of central tendency** is a single value used to describe or represent a set of data. Three common measures of central tendency are mean, median, and mode. A **measure of spread** is a value used to describe the dispersion of data. The simplest measure of spread is range.

A **mean** is an average. The mean is computed by adding all the data and dividing by the number of data points.

The **median** of a set of data is the middle number when the data is ranked (put in order). A data set with an even number of data points will have two numbers in the middle. When that is the case, the median is the mean of those two numbers.

The **range** of a set of data is the difference between the greatest and the least values in the set.

15. Zoe has 6 tests in her chemistry class. Her scores were 75, 62, 78, 92, 83, and 90. What are the mean, median, and range of her test scores?

Answer:

To find the mean, add her scores and divide by 6:

75 + 62 + 78 + 92 + 83 + 90 = 480

$\frac{480}{6}$ = **80**

To find the median, put the scores in order and find the middle term:

From smallest to largest, the data is 62, 75, 78, 83, 90, 92.

The two middle numbers are 78 and 83.

$\frac{78 + 83}{2}$ = **80.5**

To find the range of Zoe's test scores, subtract the lowest score from the highest score:

92 − 62 = **30**

Units

The United States uses customary units, sometimes called **standard units**. In this system, there are a number of different units that can be used to describe the same variable. These units and the relationships between them are shown in Table 2.4.

Table 2.4. US Customary Units		
Variable Measured	**Unit**	**Conversions**
Length	inches, foot, yard, mile	12 inches = 1 foot 3 feet = 1 yard 5,280 feet = 1 mile
Weight	ounces, pound, ton	16 ounces = 1 pound 2,000 pounds = 1 ton
Volume	fluid ounces, cup, pint, quart, gallon	8 fluid ounces = 1 cup 2 cups = 1 pint 2 pints = 1 quart 4 quarts = 1 gallon
Time	second, minute, hour, day	60 seconds = 1 minute 60 minutes = 1 hour 24 hours = 1 day
Area	square inch, square foot, square yard	144 square inches = 1 square foot 9 square feet = 1 square yard

Most other countries use the metric system, which has its own set of units for variables like length, weight, and volume. These units are modified by prefixes that make large and small numbers easier to handle. These units and prefixes are shown in Table 2.5.

Table 2.5. Metric Units and Prefixes	
Variable Measured	**Base Unit**
length	meter
weight	gram
volume	liter

Metric Prefix	**Conversion**
kilo	base unit × 1,000
hecto	base unit × 100
deka	base unit × 10
deci	base unit × 0.1
centi	base unit × 0.01
milli	base unit × 0.001

Helpful Hint: Although the United States uses the customary system, many metric units are commonly used in medical settings, including the kilogram (kg) and milliliter (mL).

Conversion factors are used to convert one unit to another (either within the same system or between different systems). A conversion factor is simply a fraction built from two equivalent values. For example, there are 12 inches in 1 foot, so the conversion factor can be $\frac{12\,in}{1\,ft}$ or $\frac{1\,ft}{12\,in}$.

To convert from one unit to another, multiple the original value by a conversion factor that has the old and new units.

How many inches are in 6 feet?

$$6\,ft \times \frac{12\,in}{1\,ft} = \frac{6\,ft \times 12\,in}{1\,ft} = 72\,in$$

PRACTICE QUESTIONS

16. How many centimeters are in 2.5 m?

Answer:

Use a conversion factor to convert centimeters to meters.

$$2.5\,m \times \frac{100\,cm}{1\,m} = \frac{2.5\,m \times 100\,cm}{1\,m} = \mathbf{250\ cm}$$

17. A newborn baby will consume 4 ounces of milk per meal and eats 6 times a day. If the baby's mother is storing the milk in pints, how many pints will she need in a week?

<u>Answer:</u>

Find the total number of ounces the baby will consume in a week.

4 oz × 6 meals a day × 7 days = 168 oz

Use a conversion factor to convert ounces to pints.

$$168 \text{ oz} \times \frac{1 \text{ cu}}{8 \text{ oz}} \times \frac{1 \text{ pt}}{2 \text{ cu}} = \textbf{10.5 pt}$$

Test Your Knowledge

Work the problem, and then choose the correct answer.

1.   65 − 14.46 + 5.8 =

   a. 14.53   b. 15.69   c. 44.74   d. 56.34   e. 73.66

2.   4.368 ÷ 2.8 =

   a. 0.0156   b. 0.156   c. 1.56   d. 15.6   e. 156

3.   Find the product of 0.4 and 0.2.

   a. 0.006   b. 0.06   c. 0.08   d. 0.6   e. 0.8

4.   Noah and Jennifer have a total of $10.00 to spend on lunch. If each buys his or her own order of french fries and a soda, how many orders of chicken strips can they share?

Menu	
Item	**Price**
Hamburger	$4.00
Chicken Strips	$4.00
Onion Rings	$3.00
French Fries	$2.00
Soda	$1.00
Shake	$1.00

   a. 0   b. 1   c. 2   d. 3   e. 4

5.   A fruit stand sells apples, bananas, and oranges at a ratio of 3:2:1. If the fruit stand sells 20 bananas, how many total pieces of fruit does the fruit stand sell?

   a. 10   b. 30   c. 40   d. 50   e. 60

6.   Juan plans to spend 25% of his workday writing a report. If he is at work for 9 hours, how many hours will he spend writing the report?

   a. 2.25   b. 2.50   c. 2.75   d. 3.25   e. 4.00

7.   John's rain gauge recorded rain on three consecutive days: $\frac{1}{2}$ in on Sunday, $\frac{2}{3}$ in on Monday, and $\frac{1}{4}$ in on Tuesday. What was the total amount of rain received over the three days?

   a. $\frac{4}{9}$ in   b. $\frac{17}{36}$ in   c. $1\frac{5}{12}$ in   d. $1\frac{1}{2}$ in   e. $1\frac{2}{3}$ in

8.   A woman's dinner bill is $48.30. If she adds a 20% tip, what will she pay in total?

   a. $9.66   b. $28.98   c. $38.64   d. $57.96   e. $68.30

9. Frank and Josh need 1 lb of chocolate to bake a cake. If Frank has $\frac{3}{8}$ lb of chocolate, and Josh has $\frac{1}{2}$ lb, how much more chocolate do they need?

a. $\frac{1}{10}$ lb b. $\frac{1}{8}$ lb c. $\frac{3}{5}$ lb d. $\frac{7}{8}$ lb e. $\frac{9}{10}$ lb

10. Students in a biology class get the following scores on a test: 97, 83, 81, 70, 64, 92, 87 What was the average score?

a. 64 b. 71 c. 82 d. 92 e. 96

ANSWER KEY

1. **d.**

Line up the decimals and subtract.

$$65.00$$
$$- 14.46$$
$$50.54$$

Line up the decimals and add.

$$50.54$$
$$+ 5.80$$
$$\mathbf{56.34}$$

2. **c.**

$4.368 \div 2.8 = \mathbf{1.56}$

3. **c.**

$0.4 \times 0.2 = \mathbf{0.08}$

4. **b.**

Write an expression to find the number of chicken strips they can afford:

$\$10 - 2(\$2.00 + \$1.00)$
$= \$10 - 2(\$3.00)$
$= \$10 - \$6.00 = \$4.00$

Four dollars is enough money to buy **one order** of chicken strips to share.

5. **e.**

Assign variables and write the ratios as fractions. Then, cross multiply to solve for the number of apples and oranges sold.

$\dfrac{\text{apples}}{\text{bananas}} = \dfrac{3}{2} = \dfrac{x}{20}$

$60 = 2x$

$x = 30$ apples

$\dfrac{\text{oranges}}{\text{bananas}} = \dfrac{1}{2} = \dfrac{y}{20}$

$2y = 20$

$y = 10$ oranges

To find the total, add the number of apples, oranges, and bananas together.

$30 + 20 + 10 = \mathbf{60\ pieces\ of\ fruit}$

6. **a.**

Use the equation for percentages.

part = whole × percentage =
$9 \times 0.25 = \mathbf{2.25}$

7. **c.**

$\dfrac{1}{2} + \dfrac{2}{3} + \dfrac{1}{4}$

$\dfrac{6}{12} + \dfrac{8}{12} + \dfrac{3}{12} = \dfrac{17}{12} = \mathbf{1\dfrac{5}{12}\ in}$

8. **d.**

Multiply the total bill by 0.2 (20%) to find the amount of the tip. Then add the tip to the total.

$\$48.30 \times 0.2 = \$9.66$
$\$48.30 + \$9.66 = \mathbf{\$57.96}$

9 **b.**

$\dfrac{3}{8} + \dfrac{1}{2} = \dfrac{3}{8} + \dfrac{4}{8} = \dfrac{7}{8}$

$1 - \dfrac{7}{8} = \dfrac{8}{8} - \dfrac{7}{8} = \mathbf{\dfrac{1}{8}\ lb}$

10. **c.**

Add the scores and divide by 7:

$\dfrac{97 + 83 + 81 + 70 + 64 + 92 + 87}{7} = \dfrac{574}{7}$

$= \mathbf{82}$

THREE: NONVERBAL SUBTEST

The twenty-five nonverbal questions on the Academic Aptitude test will gauge your spatial visualization and reasoning skills. You will be shown an analogy built from basic shapes, and you will need to select from the five answer choices to complete the analogy.

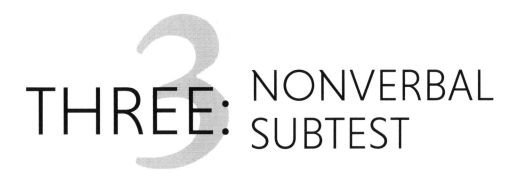

Nonverbal Question Format

Which shape correctly completes the statement?

○ is to ○ as ☐ is to ?

a.○ b.☐ c.△ d.☐ e.◇

What is an Analogy?

An **analogy** presents two sets of words or objects that share a relationship. The relationship is set up using the format

_____ is to _____ as _____ is to _____

Let's start with an example that uses words instead of shapes.

BIRD is to FLOCK as WOLF is to PACK

In this analogy, the first word is an individual animal, and the second word represents a group of those animals. A group of birds is a flock, and a group of wolves is a pack.

Solving analogies requires you to determine the relationship between the first two words, and then use that relationship to fill in the missing word:

SAIL is to BOAT as FLY is to_____

Here, the missing word is *plane*: you sail on a boat and fly on a plane.

Nonverbal Analogies

The nonverbal questions on the test will be in this same format, but they will use shapes instead of words. To answer these questions, you should look for the common relationships between the first two shapes.

ROTATING SHAPES

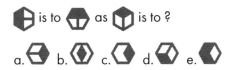

The first shape is rotated 90 degrees clockwise to give the second shape. To find the missing shape, rotate the cube 90 degrees clockwise as well.

ADDING TO SHAPES

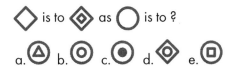

To create the second shape, another diamond is added inside the first. To find the missing shape, add another circle inside the first one.

SUBTRACTING FROM SHAPES

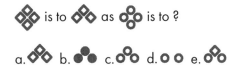

The bottom diamond is removed from the first shape to create the second. To find the missing shape, remove the bottom circle.

COMBINATIONS

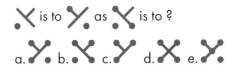

In this question, the first shape is reflected horizontally (as if shown in a mirror). Then, another circle is added to the end of the top line. To find the missing shape, reflect the given shape and add a circle to the end of the top line.

Test Your Knowledge

Which shape correctly completes the statement?

1. ◓ is to ◑ as ◒ is to ?

   a. ● b. ◐ c. ◓ d. ◑ e. ○

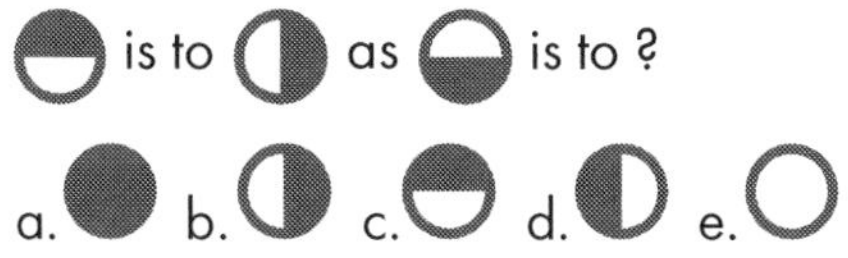

2. △ is to ☐ as ⬠ is to ?

   a. ◹ b. ▭ c. ⬡ d. ○ e. ◇

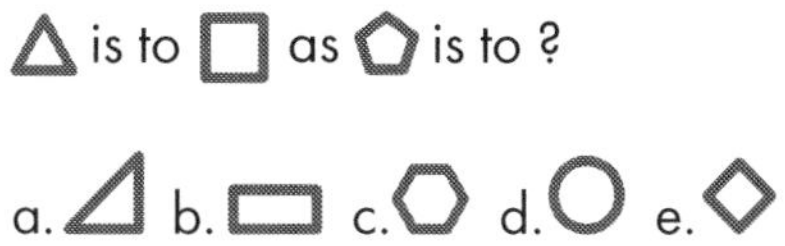

3. | is to ┬ as ╫ is to ?

   a. ╪ b. ≣ c. ☐ d. ╪ e. ┼

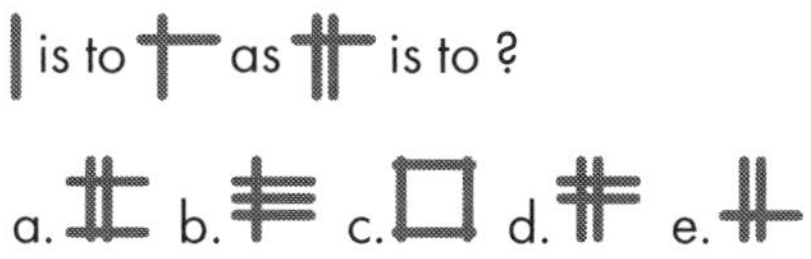

4. ⬠ is to ◇ as ◁ is to ?

   a. △ b. ▭ c. ◿ d. ◁ e. ▽

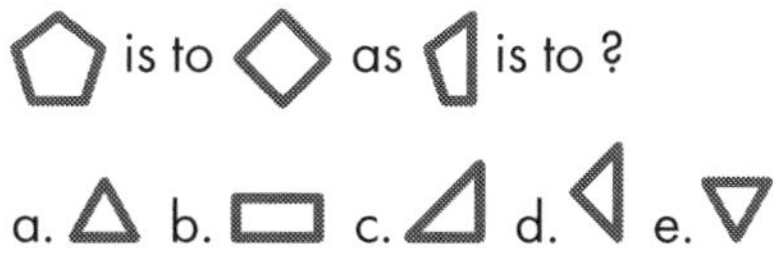

5. ❖ is to ❖ as ❖ is to ?

   a. ❖ b. ❖ c. ❖ d. ❖ e. ❖

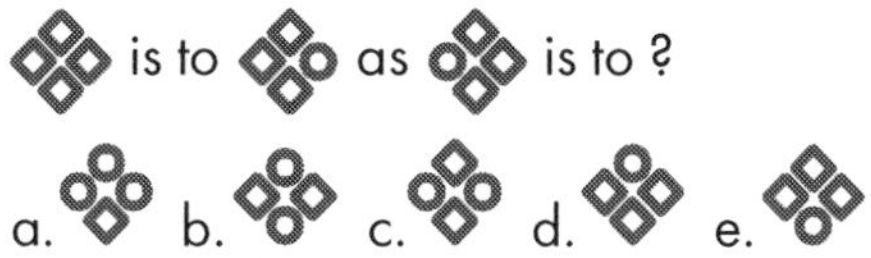

6. �III is to ⅢI as IIII is to ?

   a. ⅢⅢ b. ⅢⅢ c. ⅢⅢ d. ⅢⅢ e. ⅢⅢ

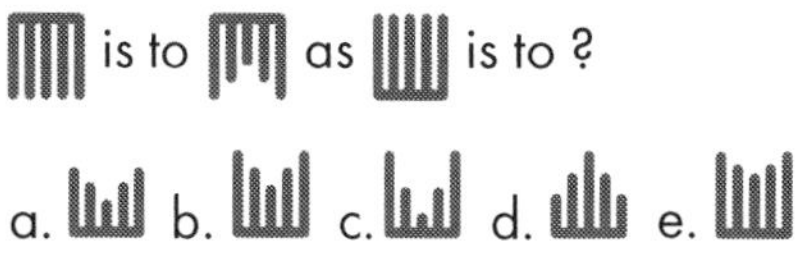

7. ◹ is to ◹ as ◹ is to ?

   a. ◹ b. ◹ c. ◹ d. ◹ e. ◹

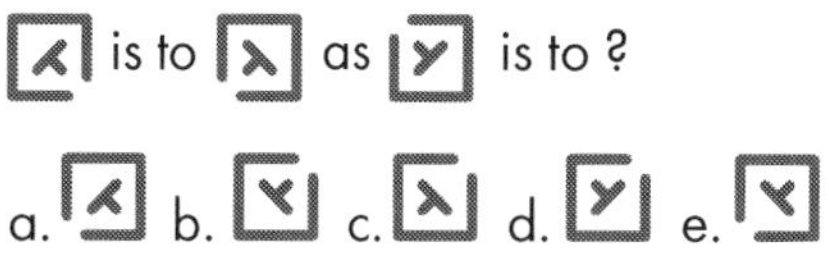

8. ❜ is to ❜ as ❜ is to ?

   a. ❜ b. ❜ c. ❜ d. ❜ e. ❜

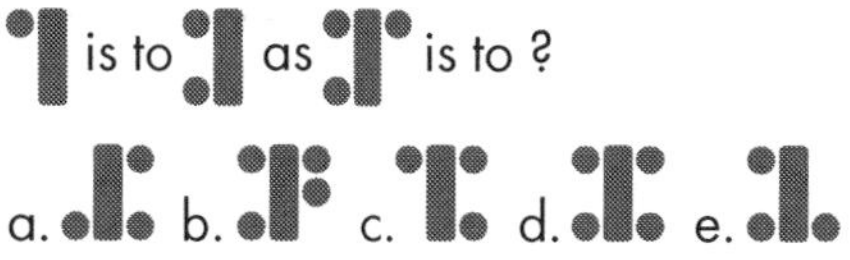

9. ⌐ is to | as ∪ is to ?

   a. ⌐ b. ⊏ c. || d. = e. ⊓

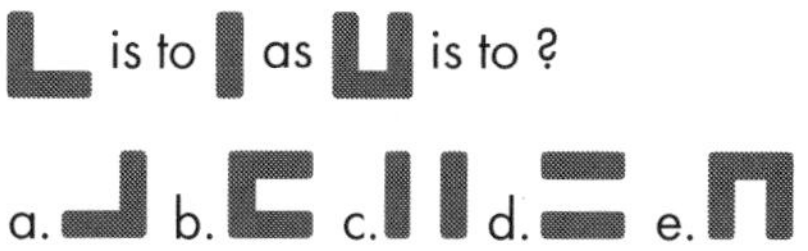

10. ⌐ is to ⌐ as ⌐ is to ?

    a. ⌐ b. ⌐ c. ⌐ d. ⌐ e. ⌐

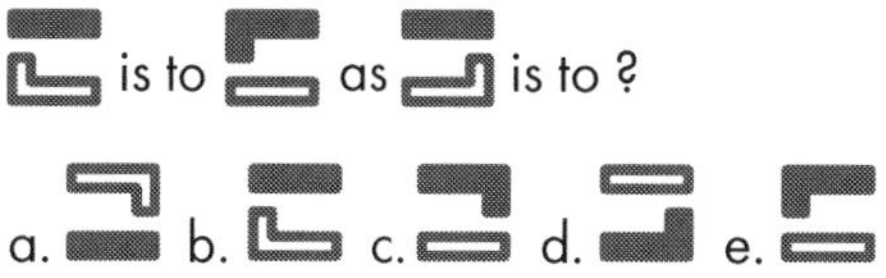

ANSWER KEY

1. **d.**

   Rotate the first shape 90 degrees clockwise to create the second shape.

2. **c.**

   Add one side to the first shape to create the second shape.

3. **d.**

   Add a horizontal line to the first shape to create the second shape.

4. **d.**

   Cut the first shape in half horizontally to create the second shape.

5. **c.**

   Change the right diamond to a circle in the first shape to create the second shape.

6. **b.**

   Shorten the inside lines of the first shape to create the second shape.

7. **b.**

   The second shape is a horizontal reflection of the first shape.

8. **d.**

   Add a circle to the side that has one circle on the first shape to create the second shape.

9. **c.**

   Remove the bottom bar from the first shape to create the second shape.

10. **a.**

   Reflect the first shape vertically and reverse the shading to create the second shape.

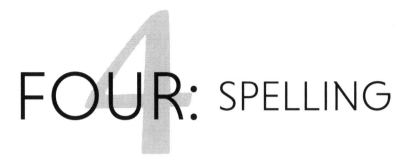

FOUR: SPELLING

The forty-five spelling questions will test your ability to pick out the correct spelling of a word from a list of three choices.

> **Spelling Question Format**
>
> *Each line below contains a word with three different spellings. Select the word from each line that is spelled correctly.*
>
> **1.**   a. intense b. intinse c. entense

As with the verbal questions, a large vocabulary will help you on this section. But when you encounter words you're not familiar with, it will help to know some basic spelling rules. You can also study the list of commonly misspelled words included at the end of this chapter.

Spelling Rule One: Plurals

Regular nouns are made plural by adding *s*. Irregular nouns can follow many different rules for pluralization, which are summarized in Table 4.1.

Table 4.1. Irregular Plural Nouns

Ends with...	Make it plural by...	Example
y	changing *y* to *i* and adding –*es*	baby → babies
f	changing *f* to *v* and adding –*es*	leaf → leaves
fe	changing *f* to *v* and adding –*s*	knife → knives
us	changing *us* to *i*	nucleus → nuclei
ch, o, s, sh, x, z	adding –*es*	catch → catches potato → potatoes pass → passes push → pushes annex → annexes blitz → blitzes

Table 4.1. Irregular Plural Nouns (continued)

Always the same	Doesn't follow the rules
sheep	man → men
deer	child → children
fish	person → people
moose	tooth → teeth
pants	goose → geese
binoculars	mouse → mice
scissors	ox → oxen

Spelling Rule Two: Conjugating Verbs

The suffixes *–ed* or *–ing* added to a regular verb generally signify the verb's tense. However, there are some exceptions to the general rule for conjugating regular verbs.

When verbs end with a silent *–e*, drop the *e* before adding *–ed* or *–ing*.

> fake → faked → faking
>
> ache → ached → aching

When verbs end in the letters *–ee*, do not drop the second *e*. Instead, simply add *–d* or *–ing*.

> free → freed → freeing
>
> agree → agreed → agreeing

When the verb ends with a single vowel plus a consonant, and the stress is at the *end* of the word, then the consonant must be doubled before adding *–ed* or *–ing*.

> commit → committed → committing
>
> refer → referred → referring

If the stress is not at the end of the word, then the consonant can remain singular.

> target → targeted → targeting
>
> visit → visited → visiting

Verbs that end with the letter *–c* must have the letter *k* added before receiving a suffix.

> panic → panicked → panicking

Spelling Rule Three: i before e

Generally, the letter *i* comes before the letter *e* in a word except when the *i* is preceded by the letter *c*.

> piece
>
> sal<u>ie</u>nt
>
> <u>cei</u>ling
>
> con<u>cei</u>vable

There are some notable exceptions where the letter *e* comes before the letter *i* such as:

+ words that end in *–cien*, like *proficient*
+ plural words ending in *–cies*, like *policies*
+ words with an *ay* sound, like *eight*, *vein*, or *neighbor*

 Helpful Hint: Be cautious of the rule "*i* comes before *e* except after *c*" because it has many exceptions. Your foreign neighbors weighed the iciest beige glaciers!

Spelling Rule Four: Suffixes

Change the final *–y* to an *i* when adding a suffix.

> lazy → laziest
>
> tidy → tidily

For words that end with the letters *–le*, replace the letter *e* with the letter *y*.

> subtle → subtly

Commonly Misspelled Words

Table 4.2 shows some commonly misspelled words. It outlines the word as correctly spelled, followed by tips to ensure proper spelling.

Table 4.2. Commonly Misspelled Words	
Correct Spelling	**Tip**
acceptable	has two c's and remember, you are *able* to accept
accommodate, accommodation	double up the c and *m*
acquire, acquit	add a c before *qu*
aggressive, aggression	spelled with two g's

Table 4.2. Commonly Misspelled Words (continued)

Correct Spelling	Tip
apparently	*ent*, not *ant*
appearance	ends with *−ance*, not *−ence*
assassination	two sets of double *s*, like Mississippi
basically	ends with *−ally*
beginning	add an *n* before adding the *−ing*
bizarre	spelled with one *z* and two *r*'s
calendar	ends with *−ar*, not *−er*
colleague	The second half is *league*, as in baseball; colleagues are like teammates!
completely	do not drop the *e*; ends with *−ely*
conscious	spelled with an *s* and *c* in the middle
definitely	spelled with *ite*, not *ate*
dilemma	double *m*
disappear	spelled with one *s* and two *p*'s
disappoint	spelled with one *s* and two *p*'s
discipline	spelled with an *s* and *c* in the middle; *i* instead of *a*
embarrass	double up *r* and *s*
environment	an *n* comes before the *m*
existence	ends with *−ence*
finally	spelled with two *l*'s
fluorescent	begins with *fluor−* and ends with *−scent*
foreign	*e* before *i*, an exception to the *ie* rule
foreseeable	begins with *fore−*, not *for−*
forty	begins with *for−*, not *four−*
forward	begins with *for−*, not *fo−*
further	begins with *fur−*, not *fu−*
gist	begins with *g*, not *j*
government	there is an *n* before the *m*
harass, harassment	spelled with one *r*, and two *s*'s
idiosyncrasy	ends with *−asy*, not *−acy*
incidentally	ends with *−ally*
independent	ends with *−ent*, not *−ant*
interrupt	spelled with two *r*'s

Correct Spelling	Tip
irresistible	ends with −*ible*
knowledge	remember the silent *d*
liaise, liaison	there is an *i* before and after the *a: iai*
necessary	spelled with one *c* and two *s*'s
noticeable	do not drop the *e* when adding −*able*
occasion	spelled with two *c*'s and one *s*
occurred, occurring	spelled with two *c*'s and two *r*'s
occurrence	spelled with two *c*'s and two *r*'s, and ends with −*ence*, not −*ance*
persistent	ends with −*ent*, not −*ant*
possession	two sets of double *s* like *Mississippi*
preferred, preferring	the second *r* is doubled
publicly	simply add −*ly* to the end of *public*
recommend	spelled with two *m*'s
reference	ends with −*ence*, not −*ance*
referred, referring	the second *r* is doubled
relevant	ends with −*ant*, not −*ent*
resistance	ends with −*ance*
sense	ends with −*se*
separate	spelled with *par* in the middle
siege	*i* before *e* rule
successful	double up the *c*'s and *s*'s
supersede	ends with −*sede*
surprise	begins with *sur*−, not *su*−
tendency	ends with −*ency*, not −*ancy*
tomorrow	spelled with one *m* and two *r*'s
tongue	begins with *ton*− and ends with −*gue*
unforeseen	spelled with an *e* after the *r*
unfortunately	do not drop the *e* when adding −*ly*
until	spelled with one *l* at the end
weird	*e* before *i*, an exception to the rule

Test Your Knowledge

Each line below contains a word with three different spellings. Select the word from each line that is spelled correctly.

1.	a. supervise	b. supervice	c. supirvise
2.	a. casuelty	b. casualty	c. cacualtie
3.	a. intensity	b. entensity	c. intensitie
4.	a. acelerate	b. accelarate	c. accelerate
5.	a. permenent	b. permanent	c. permanant
6.	a. abundent	b. abbundant	c. abundant
7.	a. burdan	b. burden	c. bourden
8.	a. prioritys	b. priorities	c. prioretees
9.	a. immense	b. emmense	c. emmence
10.	a. contaminate	b. contamenate	c. conntaminate
11.	a. arterys	b. arteries	c. artarys
12.	a. nutrishon	b. nutrition	c. nutretion
13.	a. accomplesh	b. acommplish	c. accomplish
14.	a. comppasion	b. compassion	c. commpasion
15.	a. courteous	b. corteous	c. curtaous

ANSWER KEY

1. a.
2. b.
3. a.
4. c.
5. b.
6. c.
7. b.
8. b.

9. a.
10. a.
11. b.
12. b.
13. c.
14. b.
15. a.

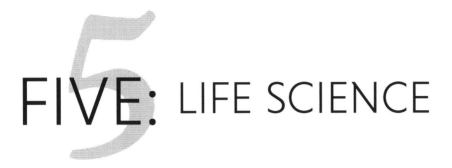

FIVE: LIFE SCIENCE

Biological Molecules

Molecules that contain carbon bound to hydrogen are **organic molecules**. Large organic molecules that contain many atoms and repeating units are **macromolecules**. Many macromolecules are **polymers** composed of repeating small units called **monomers**. There are four basic biological macromolecules that are common between all organisms: carbohydrates, lipids, proteins, and nucleic acids.

    Carbohydrates, also called sugars, are polymers made of carbon, hydrogen, and oxygen atoms. The monomer for carbohydrates are **monosaccharides**, such as glucose and fructose, that combine to form more complex sugars called **polysaccharides**. Carbohydrates store energy and provide support to cellular structures.

    Lipids, commonly known as fats, are composed mainly of hydrogen and carbon. They serve a number of functions depending on their particular structure: they make up the membrane of cells and can act as fuel, as steroids, and as hormones. Lipids are hydrophobic, meaning they repel water.

    Proteins serve an incredibly wide variety of purposes within the body. As enzymes, they play key roles in important processes like DNA replication, cellular division, and cellular metabolism. Structural proteins provide rigidity to cartilage, hair, nails, and the cytoskeletons (the network of molecules that holds the parts of a cell in place). They are also involved in communication between cells and in the transportation of molecules.

 Did You Know? An **enzyme** is a protein that accelerates a specific chemical reaction.

    Proteins are composed of individual **amino acids**, which are joined together by peptide bonds to form **polypeptides**. There are twenty amino acids, and the order of the amino acids in the polypeptide determines the shape and function of the molecule.

    Nucleic acids store hereditary information and are composed of monomers called **nucleotides**. Each nucleotide includes a sugar, a phosphate group, and a nitrogenous base.

There are two types of nucleic acids. **Deoxyribonucleic acid (DNA)** contains the genetic instructions to produce proteins. It is composed of two strings of nucleotides wound into a double helix shape. The "backbone" of the helix is made from the nucleotide's sugar (deoxyribose) and phosphate groups. The "rungs" of the ladder are made from one of four nitrogenous bases: adenine, thymine, cytosine, and guanine. These bases bond together in specific pairs: adenine with thymine and cytosine with guanine.

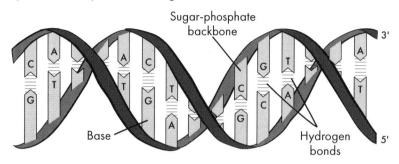

Figure 5.1. The Structure of DNA

Ribonucleic acid (RNA) transcribes information from DNA and plays several vital roles in the replication of DNA and the manufacturing of proteins. RNA nucleotides contain a sugar (ribose), a phosphate group, and one of four nitrogenous bases: adenine, uracil, cytosine, and guanine. It is usually found as a single-stranded molecule. There are three main differences between DNA and RNA:

1. DNA contains the nucleotide thymine; RNA contains the nucleotide uracil.

2. DNA is double-stranded; RNA is single-stranded.

3. DNA is made from the sugar deoxyribose; RNA is made from the sugar ribose.

PRACTICE QUESTIONS

1. The monomers that make up proteins are called
    a. monosaccharides
    b. nucleotides
    c. amino acids
    d. polypeptides
    e. enzymes

    Answer:

    c. is correct. Amino acid monomers are the building blocks of proteins.

2. Nucleic acids' primary purpose is to store
    a. carbon
    b. proteins
    c. water
    d. chemical energy
    e. genetic information

Nucleic Acids

DNA stores information by coding for proteins using blocks of three nucleotides called **codons**. Each codon codes for a specific amino acid; together, all the codons needed to make a specific protein are called a **gene**. In addition to codons for specific amino acids, there are also codons that signal "start" and "stop."

The production of a protein starts with **transcription**. During transcription, the two sides of the DNA helix unwind and a complementary strand of messenger RNA (mRNA) is manufactured using the DNA as a template.

This mRNA then travels outside the nucleus where it is "read" by a ribosome during **translation**. Each codon on the mRNA is matched to an anti-codon on a strand of tRNA, which carries a specific amino acid. The amino acids bond as they are lined up next to each other, forming a polypeptide.

When it is not being transcribed, DNA is tightly wound around proteins called **histones** to create **nucleosomes**, which are in turn packaged into **chromatin**. The structure of chromatin allows large amounts of DNA to be stored in a very small space and helps regulate transcrip-

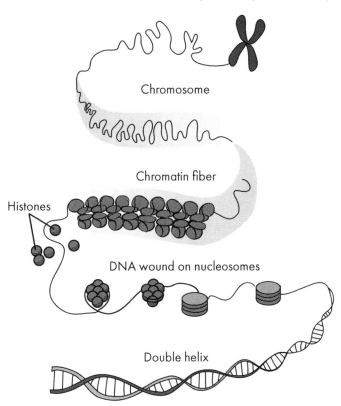

Chromosome

Chromatin fiber

Histones

DNA wound on nucleosomes

Double helix

Figure 5.2. DNA, Chromatin, and Chromosomes

tion by controlling access to specific sections of DNA. Tightly folding the DNA also helps prevent damage to the genetic code. Chromatin is further bundled into packages of DNA called **chromosomes**. During cell division, DNA is replicated to create two identical copies of each chromosome called **chromatids**.

Somatic (body) cells are **diploid**, meaning they carry two copies of each chromosome—one inherited from each parent. Gametes, which are reproductive cells, are **haploid** and carry only one copy of each chromosome. Human somatic cells have forty-six chromosomes, while human egg and sperm each carry twenty-three chromosomes.

A **mutation** causes a change in the sequence of nucleotides within DNA. For example, the codon GAC codes for the amino acid aspartic acid. However, if the cytosine is swapped for adenine, the codon now reads GAA, which corresponds to the amino acid glutamic acid. Germ-line mutations, or mutations that occur in a cell that will become a gamete, can be passed on to the offspring of an organism. Somatic mutations cannot be passed on to the offspring of an organism.

PRACTICE QUESTION

3. The information stored in RNA is used to produce a protein during

    a. replication

    b. translation

    c. transcription

    d. photosynthesis

    e. respiration

Answer:

b. is correct. Translation is the process of matching codons in RNA to the correct anti-codon to manufacture a protein.

Structure and Function of Cells

A **cell** is the smallest unit of life that can reproduce on its own. Unicellular organisms, such as amoebae, are made up of only one cell, while multicellular organisms are comprised of many cells. There are two basic types of cells: prokaryotic and eukaryotic. **Prokaryotic cells**, which include most bacteria, do not have a nucleus. The DNA in a prokaryotic cell is carried in the **cytoplasm**, which is the fluid that makes up the volume of the cell. **Eukaryotic cells** contain a nucleus where genetic material is stored.

Cells contain smaller structures called **organelles** that perform specific functions within the cell. These include **mitochondria**, which produce energy; **ribosomes**, which produce proteins; and **vacuoles**, which store water and other molecules.

Plant cells include a number of structures not found in animal cells. These include the **cell wall**, which provides the cell with a hard outer structure, and **chloroplasts**, where photo-synthesis occurs.

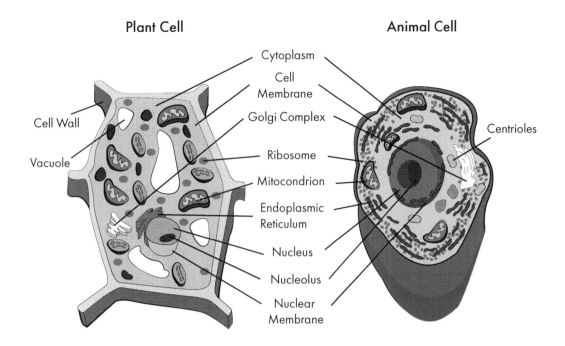

Plant Cell   Animal Cell

Cytoplasm
Cell Membrane
Golgi Complex
Ribosome
Mitocondrion
Endoplasmic Reticulum
Nucleus
Nucleolus
Nuclear Membrane

Cell Wall
Vacuole

Centrioles

Figure 5.3. Cell Organelles

The outer surface of human cells is made up of a **plasma membrane**, which gives the cell its shape. This membrane is primarily composed of a **phospholipid bilayer**, which itself is made up of two layers of lipids that face opposing directions. This functions to separate the inner cellular environment from the extracellular space, the space between cells. Molecules travel through the cell membrane using a number of different methods:

+ **Diffusion** occurs when molecules pass through the membrane from areas of high to low concentration.

+ **Facilitated diffusion** occurs with the assistance of proteins embedded in the membrane.

+ **Osmosis** is the movement of water from areas of high to low concentration.

+ During **active transport**, proteins in the membrane use energy (in the form of ATP) to move molecules across the membrane.

PRACTICE QUESTION

4. The structure that stores genetic material in a cell is the

    a.   nucleus

    b.   chloroplast

    c.   ribosome

    d.   vacuole

    e.   mitochondrion

Answer:

a. is correct. Genetic material (DNA) is stored in the nucleus.

Cellular Respiration

Organisms use chains of chemical reactions called **biochemical pathways** to acquire, store, and use energy. The molecule most commonly used to store energy is **adenosine triphosphate (ATP)**. When a phosphate group (Pi) is removed from ATP, creating **adenosine diphosphate (ADP)**, energy is released. The cell harnesses this energy to perform processes such as transport, growth, and replication.

Cells also transfer energy using the molecules **nicotinamide adenine dinucleotide phosphate (NADPH)** and **nicotinamide adenine dinucleotide (NADH)**. These molecules are generally used to carry energy-rich electrons during the process of creating ATP.

In **cellular respiration**, food molecules such as glucose are broken down, and the electrons harvested from these molecules are used to make ATP. The first stage of cellular respiration is an **anaerobic** (does not require oxygen) process called **glycolysis**. Glycolysis takes place in the cytoplasm of a cell and transforms glucose into two molecules of pyruvate. In the process, two molecules of ATP and two molecules of NADH are produced.

Under anaerobic conditions, pyruvate is reduced to acids and sometimes gases and/or alcohols in a process called **fermentation**. However, this process is less efficient than aerobic cellular respiration and produces only two ATP.

Under aerobic conditions, pyruvate enters the second stage of cellular respiration—the **Krebs cycle**. The Krebs cycle takes place in the mitochondria, or tubular organelles, of a eukaryotic cell. Here, pyruvate is oxidized completely to form six molecules of carbon dioxide (CO_2). This set of reactions also produces two more molecules of ATP, ten molecules of NADH, and two molecules of $FADH_2$ (an electron carrier).

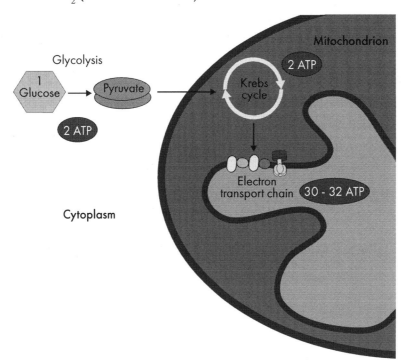

Figure 5.4. Cellular Respiration

The electrons carried by NADH and FADH$_2$ are transferred to the **electron transport chain**, where they cascade through carrier molecules embedded in the inner mitochondrial membrane. Oxygen is the final electron receptor in the chain; it reacts with these electrons and hydrogen to form water. This sequential movement of electrons drives the formation of a proton (H$^+$) gradient, which is used by the enzyme ATP synthase to produce ATP. The electron transport chain produces thirty to thirty-two molecules of ATP.

The balanced chemical equation for cellular respiration is:

$$C_6H_{12}O_6 + 6O_2 \rightarrow 6CO_2 + 6H_2O$$

PRACTICE QUESTION

5. The stage of cellular respiration that produces the largest number of ATP molecules is

    a. glycolysis

    b. fermentation

    c. the Krebs cycle

    d. the electron transport chain

    e. the citric acid cycle

    Answer:

    d. is correct. The electron transport chain produces thirty to thirty-two molecules of ATP made during cellular respiration. The other choices each produce only two molecules of ATP.

Photosynthesis

The sun powers nearly all biological systems on this planet. Plants, along with some bacteria and algae, harness the energy of sunlight and transform it into chemical energy through the process of **photosynthesis.**

Inside each chloroplast are stacks of flat, interconnected sacs called **thylakoids.** Within the membrane of each thylakoid sac are light-absorbing pigments called **chlorophyll.**

In the light-dependent reactions of photosynthesis, light penetrates the chloroplast and strikes the chlorophyll. The energy in the sunlight excites electrons, boosting them to a higher energy level. These excited electrons then cascade through the **electron transport chain,** creating energy in the form of ATP and NADPH. This reaction also splits water to release O$_2$.

The ATP and NADPH created by the light-dependent stage of photosynthesis enter the **Calvin cycle,** which uses the energy to produce the carbohydrate glucose (C$_6$H$_{12}$O$_6$). The carbon needed for this reaction comes from atmospheric CO$_2$.

The balanced chemical equation for photosynthesis is:

$$6CO_2 + 6H_2O \rightarrow C_6H_{12}O_6 + 6O_2$$

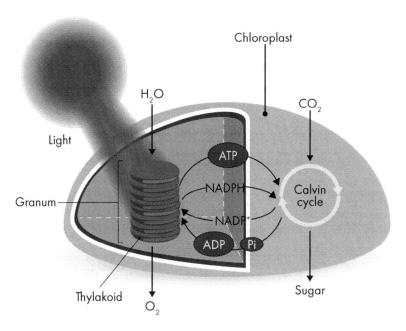

Granum

Light

Thylakoid

Figure 5.5. Photosynthesis

PRACTICE QUESTION

6. Glucose is produced during the Calvin cycle using

a. O_2

b. CO_2

c. ADP

d. H_2

e. N_2

Answer:

b. is correct. During the Calvin cycle, carbon dioxide (CO_2) is used to produce glucose.

Cell Division

The process of cell growth and reproduction is the **cell cycle**. Eukaryotic cells spend the majority of their lifespan in **interphase**, during which the cell performs necessary functions and grows. During interphase, the cell also copies its DNA. Then, during **mitosis** the two identical sets of DNA are pulled to opposite sides of the cell. The cell then splits during **cytokinesis**, resulting in two cells that have identical copies of the original cell's DNA.

Meiosis is the process of sexual reproduction, or the formation of gametes (egg and sperm cells). During meiosis, the replicated DNA is separated to form two diploid cells. These cells in turn will separate again, with each cell retaining a single set of chromosomes. The result is four haploid cells.

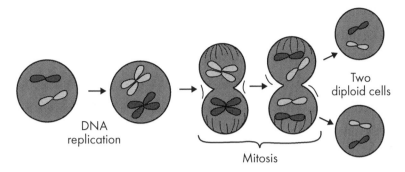

Figure 5.6. Mitosis

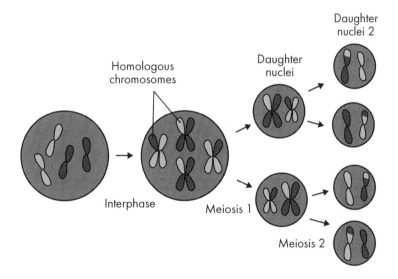

Figure 5.7. Meiosis

PRACTICE QUESTION

7.   The result of mitosis and cytokinesis is
    a.   two haploid cells
    b.   four haploid cells
    c.   eight haploid cells
    d.   two diploid cells
    e.   four diploid cells
    Answer:
    d. is correct. The daughter cells produced during mitosis are genetically identical to their diploid (2n) parent.

Genetics

Genetics is the study of heredity—how characteristics are passed from parents to offspring. These characteristics, or traits, are determined by genes. Each individual has two versions of the same gene, called **alleles**, with one contributed by each parent. An individual is **homozygous** for a particular gene if both alleles are the same, and **heterozygous** if the two alleles are different.

> 🔍 Helpful Hint: Alleles are written as a single letter with the dominant allele capitalized (A) and the recessive allele lowercase (a).

For a particular gene, the **dominant** allele will always be expressed, and the **recessive** allele will only be expressed if the other allele is also recessive. In other words, a recessive trait is only expressed if the individual is homozygous for that allele.

The full set of genetic material in an organism is its **genotype**. The organism's **phenotype** is the set of observable traits in the organism. For example, brown hair is a phenotype. The genotype of this trait is a set of alleles that contain the genetic information for brown hair.

The genotype, and resulting phenotype, of sexually reproducing organisms can be tracked using **Punnett squares**, which show the alleles of the parent generation on each of two axes. The possible genotypes of the resulting offspring, called the F1 generation, are then shown in the body of the square.

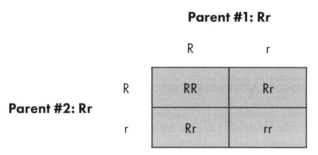

Figure 5.8. Punnett Square

In Figure 5.8., two heterozygous parents for trait R are mated, resulting in the following genotypes and phenotypes for the offspring:

✦ 1 homozygous dominant (dominant phenotype)

✦ 2 heterozygous (dominant phenotype)

✦ 1 homozygous recessive (recessive phenotype)

> 🔍 Did You Know? Many of the rules of genetics were discovered by Gregor Mendel, a nineteenth-century abbot who used pea plants to show how traits are passed down through generations.

Non-Mendelian inheritance describes patterns that do not follow the ratios described above. These patterns can occur for a number of reasons. Alleles might show **incomplete dominance**, where one allele is not fully expressed over the other, resulting in a third phenotype (for example, a red flower and white flower cross to create a pink flower). Alleles can also be **codominant**, meaning both are fully expressed (such as the AB blood type).

The expression of genes can also be regulated by mechanisms other than the dominant/recessive relationship. For example, some genes may inhibit the expression of other genes, a process called **epistasis**. The environment can also impact gene expression. For example, organisms with the same genotype may grow to different sizes depending on the nutrients available to them.

PRACTICE QUESTIONS

8. The dominant allele will not be expressed when
   a. a recessive allele from the father is paired with a recessive allele from the mother
   b. a dominant allele from the father is paired with a dominant allele from the mother
   c. a dominant allele from the father is paired with a recessive allele from the mother
   d. a recessive allele from the father is paired with a dominant allele from the mother
   e. a recessive allele from the father is paired with no allele from the mother

   Answer:

   a. is correct. This genotype is homozygous, and the recessive trait is the only trait that can be expressed.

9. Alleles for brown eyes (B) are dominant over alleles for blue eyes (b). If two parents are both heterozygous for this gene, the percent chance that their offspring will have brown eyes is
   a. 0 percent
   b. 25 percent
   c. 50 percent
   d. 75 percent
   e. 100 percent

   Answer:

   d. is correct. The Punnett square shows that there is a 75 percent chance the child will have the dominant B gene, and thus have brown eyes.

	B	**b**
B	BB	Bb
b	Bb	bb

Evolution

Evolution is the gradual genetic change in species over time. Natural selection alters the variation and frequency of certain alleles and phenotypes within a population. This increased variation and frequency leads to varying reproductive success, in which individuals with certain traits survive over others. Combined, these mechanisms lead to gradual changes in the genotype of individual populations that, over time, can result in the creation of a new species.

Natural selection is a process in which only the members of a population best adapted to their environment tend to survive and reproduce, which ensures that their favorable traits will be passed on to future generations of the species. There are four basic conditions that must be met in order for natural selection to occur:

1. inherited variation
2. overproduction of offspring
3. fitness to environment
4. differential reproduction

 Check Your Understanding: Why might a harmful mutation continue to exist in a population?

The offspring with inherited variations best suited for their environment will be more likely to survive than others and are therefore more likely to pass on their successful genes to future populations through reproduction. This is referred to as **fitness**. An organism that is considered biologically "fit" will be more successful passing on its genes through reproduction compared to other members of the population. The frequency of certain alleles in a gene pool will change as a result.

Artificial selection occurs in a species when humans get involved in the reproductive process. Over time, humans have intentionally bred organisms with the same desirable traits in a process called selective breeding. This has led to the evolution of many common crops and farm animals that are bred specifically for human consumption, as well as among domesticated animals, such as horses or dogs.

PRACTICE QUESTION

10. Natural selection is NOT occurring when
   a. peahens select the most brightly colored peacocks as mates
   b. large bears chase smaller rivals away from food sources
   c. sparrows with a certain beak shape reach plentiful food sources
   d. farmers plant seeds only from the most productive corn plants
   e. male ibex use their horns to fight other males before mating with females

   Answer:

   d. is correct. Farmers choosing specific traits in plants is an example of artificial selection.

Ecology

Ecology is the study of organisms' interactions with each other and the environment. Ecologists break down the groups of organisms and abiotic features into hierarchal groups.

Groups of organisms of the same species living in the same geographic area are called **populations**. These organisms will compete with each other for resources and mates and will display characteristic patterns in growth related to their interactions with the environment. For example, many populations exhibit a carrying capacity, which is the highest number of individuals that the resources in a given environment can support. Populations that outgrow their carrying capacity are likely to experience increased death rates until the population reaches a stable level again.

Populations of different species living together in the same geographic region are called **communities**. Within a community there are many different interactions among individuals of different species. **Predators** consume **prey** for food, and some species are in **competition** for the same limited pool of resources. In a **symbiotic** relationship, two species have evolved to share a close relationship. Two species may also have a **parasitic** relationship in which one organism benefits to the detriment of the other, such as ticks feeding off a dog. Both species benefit in a **mutualistic** relationship, and in a **commensalistic** relationship, one species benefits and the other feels the effects.

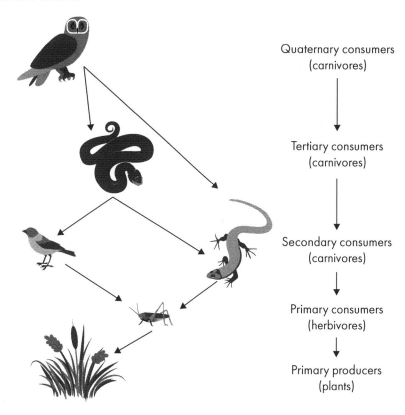

Figure 5.9. Food Web

Within a community, a species exists in a **food web**: every species either consumes or is consumed by another (or others). The lowest trophic level in the web is occupied by **producers**, which include plants and algae that produce energy directly from the sun. The next level are **primary consumers** (herbivores), which consume plant matter. The next trophic level includes **secondary consumers** (carnivores), which consume herbivores.

A food web may also contain another level of **tertiary consumers** (carnivores that consume other carnivores). In a real community, these webs can be extremely complex, with species existing on multiple trophic levels. Communities also include **decomposers**, which are organisms that break down dead matter.

The collection of biotic (living) and abiotic (nonliving) features in a geographic area is called an **ecosystem**. For example, in a forest, the ecosystem consists of all the organisms (animals, plants, fungi, bacteria, etc.), in addition to the soil, groundwater, rocks, and other abiotic features.

Biomes are collections of plant and animal communities that exist within specific climates. They are similar to ecosystems, but they do not include abiotic components and can exist within and across continents. For example, the Amazon rainforest is a specific ecosystem, while tropical rainforests in general are considered a biome that includes a set of similar communities across the world. Together, all the living and nonliving parts of the earth are known as the **biosphere**.

Terrestrial biomes are usually defined by distinctive patterns in temperature and rainfall, and aquatic biomes are defined by the type of water and organisms found there. Examples of biomes include:

+ **deserts**: extreme temperatures and very low rainfall with specialized vegetation and small mammals

+ **tropical rainforests**: hot and wet with an extremely high diversity of species

+ **temperate grasslands**: moderate precipitation and distinct seasons with grasses and shrubs dominating

+ **temperate forests**: moderate precipitation and temperatures with deciduous trees dominating

+ **tundra**: extremely low temperatures and short growing seasons with little or no tree growth

+ **coral reefs**: a marine (saltwater) system with high levels of diversity

+ **lake**: an enclosed body of fresh water

If the delicate balance of an ecosystem is disrupted, the system may not function properly. For example, if all the secondary consumers disappear, the population of primary consumers would increase, causing the primary consumers to overeat the producers and eventually starve. **Keystone species** are especially important in a particular community, and removing them decreases the overall diversity of the ecosystem.

PRACTICE QUESTIONS

11. An abiotic environmental factor that influences population size is

a. food availability

b. rate of precipitation

c. mutualism

d. competition

e. predation

Answer:

b. is correct. Precipitation is a nonliving (abiotic) factor that influences population size.

12. The terrestrial biome characterized by moderate rainfall and the dominance of deciduous trees is called

a. desert

b. tropical rainforest

c. temperate forest

d. tundra

e. grasslands

Answer:

c. is correct. Temperate forests have moderate rainfall and are dominated by deciduous trees.

Human Anatomy and Physiology

In a multicellular organism, cells are grouped together into **tissues**, and these tissues are grouped into **organs**, which perform specific **functions**. The heart, for example, is the organ that pumps blood throughout the body. Organs are further grouped into **organ systems**, such as the digestive or respiratory systems.

Anatomy is the study of the structure of organisms, and **physiology** is the study of how these structures function. Both disciplines study the systems that allow organisms to perform a number of crucial functions, including the exchange of energy, nutrients, and waste products with the environment. This exchange allows organisms to maintain **homeostasis**, or the stabilization of internal conditions.

Helpful Hint: In science, a **system** is a collection of interconnected parts that make up a complex whole with defined boundaries. Systems may be closed, meaning nothing passes in or out of them, or open, meaning they have inputs and outputs.

The human body has a number of systems that perform vital functions, including the digestive, excretory, respiratory, circulatory, skeletal, muscular, immune, nervous, endocrine, and reproductive systems.

The **digestive system** breaks food down into nutrients for use by the body's cells. Food enters through the **mouth** and moves through the **esophagus** to the **stomach**, where it is physically and chemically broken down. The food particles then move into the **small intestine**, where the majority of nutrients are absorbed. Finally, the remaining particles enter the **large intestine**, which mostly absorbs water, and waste exits through the **rectum** and **anus**. This system also includes other organs, such as the **liver**, **gallbladder**, and **pancreas**, that manufacture substances needed for digestion.

The **genitourinary system** removes waste products from the body. Its organs include the liver, which breaks down harmful

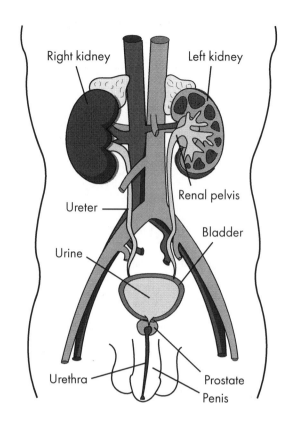

Figure 5.10. Genitourinary System

substances, and the **kidneys**, which filter waste from the bloodstream. The excretory system also includes the **bladder** and **urinary tract**, which expel the waste filtered by the kidneys;

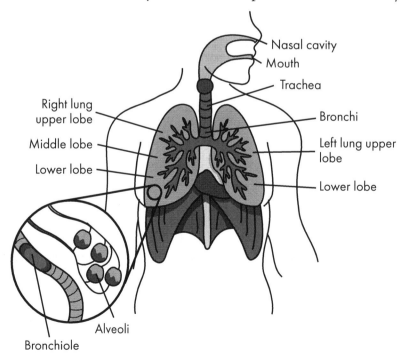

Figure 5.11. Respiratory System

the lungs, which expel the carbon dioxide created by cellular metabolism; and the skin, which secretes salt in the form of perspiration.

The **respiratory system** takes in oxygen (which is needed for cellular functioning) and expels carbon dioxide. Humans take in air primarily through the nose but also through the mouth. This air travels down the **trachea** and **bronchi** into the **lungs**, which are composed of millions of small structures called alveoli that allow for the exchange of gases between the blood and the air.

The circulatory system carries oxygen, nutrients, and waste products in the blood to and from all the cells of the body. The **heart** is a four-chambered muscle that pumps blood throughout the body. The four chambers are the right atrium, right ventricle, left atrium, and left ventricle. Deoxygenated blood (blood from which all the oxygen has been extracted and used) enters the right atrium and then is sent from the right ventricle through the pulmonary artery to the lungs, where it collects oxygen. The oxygen-rich blood then returns to the left atrium of the heart and is pumped out the left ventricle to the rest of the body.

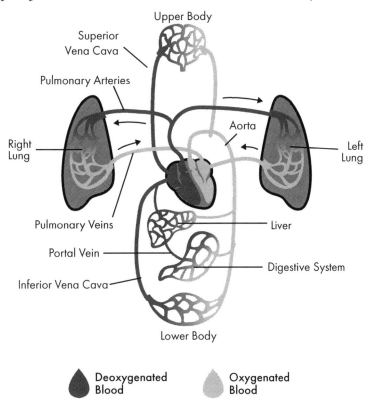

Figure 5.12. Circulatory System

Blood travels through a system of vessels. **Arteries** branch directly off the heart and carry blood away from it. The largest artery is the aorta, which carries blood from the heart to the rest of the body. **Veins** carry blood back to the heart from other parts of the body. Most veins carry deoxygenated blood, but the pulmonary veins carry oxygenated blood from the lungs back to the heart to then be pumped to the rest of the body. Arteries and veins branch into smaller and smaller vessels until they become **capillaries**, which are the smallest vessels and the site where gas exchange occurs.

The **skeletal system**, which is composed of the body's **bones** and **joints**, provides support for the body and helps with movement. Bones also store some of the body's nutrients and produce specific types of cells. Humans are born with 237 bones. However, many of these bones fuse during childhood, and adults have only 206 bones. Bones can have a rough or smooth texture and come in four basic shapes: long, flat, short, and irregular.

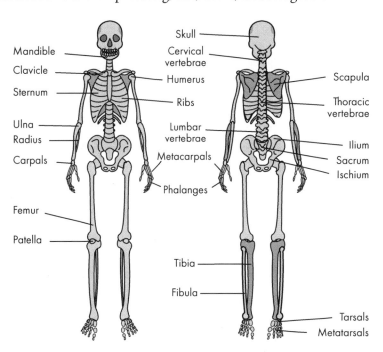

Figure 5.13. The Skeletal System

The **muscular system** allows the body to move and also moves blood and other substances through the body. The human body has three types of muscles. Skeletal muscles are voluntary muscles (meaning they can be controlled) that are attached to bones and move the body. Smooth muscles are involuntary muscles (meaning they cannot be controlled) that create movement in parts of the digestive tract, blood vessels, and the reproduction system. Finally, cardiac muscle is the involuntary muscle that contracts the heart, pumping blood throughout the body.

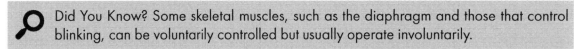

Did You Know? Some skeletal muscles, such as the diaphragm and those that control blinking, can be voluntarily controlled but usually operate involuntarily.

The **immune system** protects the body from infection by foreign particles and organisms. It includes the **skin** and mucous membranes, which act as physical barriers, and a number of specialized cells that destroy foreign substances in the body. The human body has an adaptive immune system, meaning it can recognize and respond to foreign substances once it has been exposed to them. This is the underlying mechanism behind vaccines.

The immune system is composed of **B cells**, or B lymphocytes, that produce special proteins called **antibodies** that bind to foreign substances, called **antigens**, and neutralize them. **T cells**, or T lymphocytes, remove body cells that have been infected by foreign invaders like bacteria or viruses. **Helper T cells** coordinate production of antibodies by B cells and removal of infected cells by T cells. **Killer T cells** destroy body cells that have been infected by invaders after they are identified and removed by T cells. Finally, **memory cells** remember antigens that have been removed so the immune system can respond more quickly if they enter the body again.

> Did You Know? Memory B cells are the underlying mechanisms behind vaccines, which introduce a harmless version of a pathogen into the body to activate the body's adaptive immune response.

The **nervous system** processes external stimuli and sends signals throughout the body. It is made up of two parts. The central nervous system (CNS) includes the brain and spinal cord and is where information is processed and stored. The brain has three parts: the cerebrum, cerebellum, and medulla. The **cerebrum** is the biggest part of the brain, the wrinkly gray part at the front and top, and controls different functions like thinking, vision, hearing, touch, and smell. The **cerebellum** is located at the back and bottom of the brain and controls motor movements. The **medulla**, or brain stem, is where the brain connects to the spinal cord and controls automatic body functions like breathing and heartbeat.

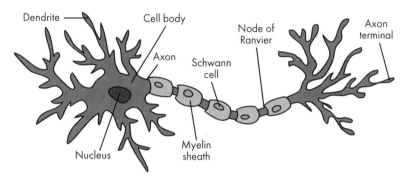

Figure 5.14. Neuron

The peripheral nervous system (PNS) includes small cells called **neurons** that transmit information throughout the body using electrical signals. Neurons are made up of three basic parts: the cell body, dendrites, and axons. The cell body is the main part of the cell where the organelles are located. Dendrites are long arms that extend from the main cell body and communicate with other cells' dendrites through chemical messages passed across a space called a synapse. Axons are extensions from the cell body and transmit messages to the muscles.

The **endocrine system** is a collection of organs that produce **hormones**, which are chemicals that regulate bodily processes. These organs include the pituitary gland, hypothalamus, pineal gland, thyroid gland, parathyroid glands, adrenal glands, testes (in males), ovaries (in females), and the placenta (in pregnant females). Together, the hormones these organs produce regulate a wide variety of bodily functions, including hunger, sleep, mood, reproduction, and temperature. Some organs that are part of other systems can also act as endocrine organs, including the pancreas and liver.

The reproductive system includes the organs necessary for sexual reproduction. In males, sperm is produced in the **testes** (also known as **testicles**) and carried through a thin tube called the **vas deferens** to the **urethra**, which carries sperm through the **penis** and out of the body.

The **prostate** is a muscular gland approximately the size of a walnut that is located between the male bladder and penis and produces a fluid that nourishes and protects sperm.

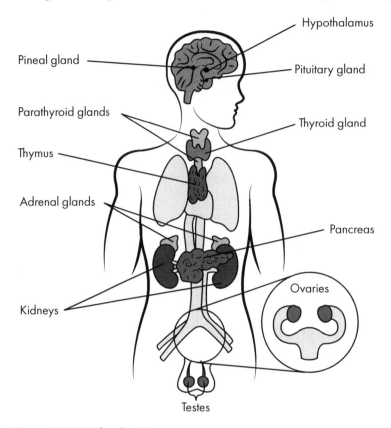

Figure 5.15. Endocrine System

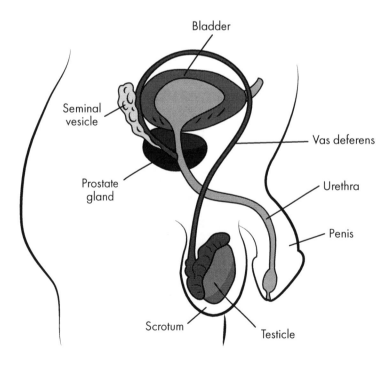

Figure 5.16. Male Reproductive System

In the female reproductive system, eggs are produced in the **ovaries** and released roughly once a month to move through the **fallopian tubes** to the **uterus**. If an egg is fertilized, the new embryo implants in the lining of the uterus and develops over the course of about nine months. At the end of **gestation**, the baby leaves the uterus through the cervix, and exits the body through the **vagina**. If the egg is not fertilized, the uterus will shed its lining.

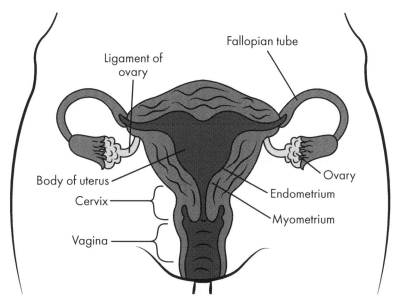

Figure 5.17. Female Reproductive System

PRACTICE QUESTIONS

13.   The small bones in the hands are known as the

   a.   tarsals

   b.   ribs

   c.   metatarsals

   d.   vertebrae

   e.   phalanges

   Answer:

   e. is correct. The small bones in the fingers of the hands are the phalanges.

14.   In the digestive tract, most of the nutrients are absorbed in the

   a.   small intestine

   b.   rectum

   c.   stomach

   d.   large intestine

   e.   esophagus

   Answer:

   a. is correct. Most nutrients are absorbed by the small intestine.

Test Your Knowledge

Read the question, and then choose the most correct answer.

1. Which of the following is NOT a nucleobase of DNA?

   a. adenine

   b. guanine

   c. thymine

   d. uracil

2. Which of the following is a monomer used to build carbohydrates?

   a. glucose

   b. thymine

   c. aspartic acid

   d. histone

3. Which of the following processes uses the information stored in RNA to produce a protein?

   a. replication

   b. translation

   c. transcription

   d. mutation

4. The information stored in DNA is used to make which of the following molecules?

   a. amino acids

   b. proteins

   c. fatty acids

   d. monosaccharides

5. Which of the following is NOT present in an animal cell?

   a. nucleus

   b. mitochondria

   c. cytoplasm

   d. cell wall

6. Which of the following cell organelles are the site of lipid synthesis?

   a. smooth endoplasmic reticulum

   b. ribosome

   c. rough endoplasmic reticulum

   d. Golgi apparatus

7. Which of the following cellular processes does NOT use ATP?

   a. facilitated diffusion

   b. DNA replication

   c. active transport through the cell membrane

   d. movement of the mot complex in a flagellum

8. Which of the following molecules can be found in abundance in a fatigued muscle?

   a. glucose

   b. lactic acid

   c. ATP

   d. myoglobin

9. Why do some photosynthetic structures, like leaves, appear green?

   a. The epidermis of the leaf absorbs red and blue light.

   b. The epidermis of the leaf absorbs green light.

   c. The chlorophyll of the leaf absorbs red and blue light.

   d. The chlorophyll of the leaf absorbs green light.

10. The Calvin cycle produces one molecule of glucose from which of the following three molecules?
    a. ATP, NADPH, and O_2
    b. ATP, NADPH, and CO_2
    c. CO_2, H_2O, and ATP
    d. CO_2, H_2O, and O_2

11. The result of meiosis and cytokinesis is
    a. two haploid (1n) cells.
    b. four haploid (1n) cells.
    c. two diploid (2n) cells.
    d. four diploid (2n) cells.

12. Alleles for brown eyes (B) are dominant over alleles for blue eyes (b). If two parents are both heterozygous for this gene, what is the percent chance that their offspring will have brown eyes?
    a. 25
    b. 50
    c. 75
    d. 100

13. If a plant that is homozygous dominant (T) for a trait is crossed with a plant that is homozygous recessive (t) for the same trait, what will be the phenotype of the offspring if the trait follows Mendelian patterns of inheritance?
    a. All offspring will show the dominant phenotype.
    b. All offspring will show the recessive phenotype.
    c. Half the offspring will show the dominant trait, and the other half will show the recessive phenotype.
    d. All the offspring will show a mix of the dominant and recessive phenotypes.

14. A female who carries the recessive color blindness gene mates with a color-blind male, resulting in a male child. Which of the following numbers represents the likelihood the offspring will also be color blind?
    a. 25 percent
    b. 50 percent
    c. 100 percent
    d. 0 percent

15. Type AB blood—the expression of both A and B antigens on a red blood cell surface—occurs as the result of which of the following?
    a. incomplete dominance
    b. recombination
    c. codominance
    d. independent assortment

16. Which of the following is NOT a condition of natural selection?
    a. differential reproduction
    b. competition between species
    c. overproduction of offspring
    d. inheritance of traits

17. Which of the following is the type of nonrandom mating that leads to changes in allele frequency?
    a. sexual selection
    b. genetic drift
    c. migration
    d. gene flow

18. Which of the following aquatic biomes are located where freshwater streams empty into the ocean?
    a. wetlands
    b. coral reef
    c. estuaries
    d. littoral

19. Which of the following scenarios accurately describes primary succession?

   a. The ground is scorched by a lava flow; later the establishment of lichens begins on the volcanic rock, leading to the eventual formation of soils.

   b. A meadow is destroyed by a flood; eventually small grasses begin to grow again to begin establishing a healthy meadow ecosystem.

   c. A fire destroys a section of a forest; once the ashes clear, small animals begin making their homes within the area.

   d. A farmer overuses the land causing all the minerals and nutrients in the soil to be used up. Some leftover grass seeds in the soil begin to sprout, repopulating the land.

20. A barnacle is attached to the outside of the whale to collect and consume particulate matter as the whale moves through the ocean. The barnacle benefits, while the whale is unaffected. The phenomenon described is an example of

   a. predation

   b. commensalism

   c. mutualism

   d. parasitism

21. Which of the following organisms generate their own food through photosynthesis and make up the first level of the energy pyramid?

   a. heterotrophs

   b. autotrophs

   c. producers

   d. consumers

22. Which of the following is composed only of members of the same species?

   a. ecosystem

   b. community

   c. biome

   d. population

23. Which of the following type of muscle is responsible for voluntary movement in the body?

   a. cardiac

   b. visceral

   c. smooth

   d. skeletal

24. Which of the following organs is an accessory organ that food does NOT pass through as part of digestion?

   a. pharynx

   b. mouth

   c. small intestine

   d. liver

25. Which of the following is NOT a function of the respiratory system in humans?

   a. to exchange gas

   b. to produce sound and speech

   c. to distribute oxygen to the rest of the body

   d. to remove particles from the air

ANSWER KEY

1. **d.**

Uracil (U) is a pyrimidine found in RNA, replacing the thymine (T) pyrimidine found in DNA.

2. **a.**

Glucose is a monosaccharide that can be used to build larger polysaccharides.

3. **b.**

Translation is a process of matching codons in RNA to the correct anti-codon to manufacture a protein.

4. **b.**

Proteins are the expressed products of a gene.

5. **d.**

The cell wall is the structure that gives plant cells their rigidity.

6. **a.**

The smooth endoplasmic reticulum is a series of membranes attached to the cell nucleus and plays an important role in the production and storage of lipids. It is called smooth because it lacks ribosomes on the membrane surface.

7. **a.**

Facilitated diffusion is a form of passive transport across the cell membrane and does not use energy.

8. **b.**

Lactic acid, a byproduct of anaerobic respiration, builds up in muscles and causes fatigue. This occurs when the energy exerted by the muscle exceeds the amount of oxygen available for aerobic respiration.

9. **c.**

Light passes through the epidermis and strikes the pigment chlorophyll, which absorbs the wavelengths of light that humans see as red and blue and reflects the wavelengths of light that the human eye perceives as green.

10. **b.**

Glucose is produced from CO_2 by the energy stored in ATP and the hydrogen atoms associated with NADPH.

11. **b.**

Four haploid (1n) cells are produced during meiosis.

12. **c.**

The Punnett square shows that there is a 75 percent chance the child will have the dominant B gene, and thus have brown eyes.

	B	b
B	BB	Bb
b	Bb	bb

13. **a.**

Because each offspring will inherit the dominant allele, all the offspring will show the dominant phenotype. The offspring would only show a mix of the two phenotypes if they did not follow Mendelian inheritance patterns.

14. **b.**

The offspring has a 50 percent chance of inheriting the dominant allele and a 50 percent chance of inheriting the recessive allele from his mother.

15. **c.**

Type AB blood occurs when two equally dominant alleles (A and B) are inherited. Since they are both dominant, one does not mask the other; instead, both are expressed.

16. **b.**

Competition between species is not necessary for natural selection to occur, although it can influence the traits that are selected for within a population.

17. **a.**

Sexual selection changes allele frequency because it leads to some members of the population reproducing more frequently than others.

18. **c.**

Estuaries are found at the boundary of ocean and stream biomes and are very ecologically productive areas.

19. **a.**

Primary succession can only occur on newly exposed earth that was not previously inhabited by living things. Often this new land is the result of lava flows or glacial movement.

20. **b.**

In a commensal relationship, one species benefits with no impact on the other.

21. **c.**

Producers are a kind of autotroph that are found on the energy pyramid and produce food via photosynthesis.

22. **d.**

A population is all the members of the same species in a given area.

23. **d.**

Skeletal muscles are attached to the skeletal system and are controlled voluntarily.

24. **d.**

The liver is an accessory organ that detoxifies ingested toxins and produces bile for fat digestion.

25. **c.**

The cardiovascular system distributes oxygen to the rest of the body.

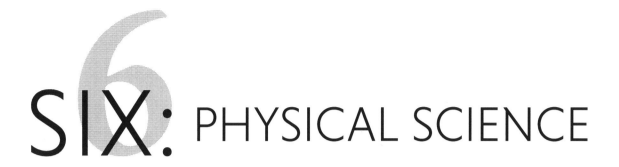

SIX: PHYSICAL SCIENCE

The Structure of the Atom

All matter is composed of very small particles called **atoms**. Atoms can be further broken down into subatomic particles. **Protons**, which are positive, and **neutrons**, which are neutral, form the nucleus of the atom. Negative particles called **electrons** orbit the nucleus.

While electrons are often depicted as orbiting the nucleus like a planet orbits the sun, they're actually arranged in cloud-like areas called **shells**. The shells closest to the nucleus have the lowest energy and are filled first. The high-energy shells farther from the nucleus only fill with electrons once lower-energy shells are full.

The outermost electron shell of an atom is its **valence shell**. The electrons in this shell are involved in chemical reactions. Atoms are most stable when their valence shell is full (usually with eight electrons), so the atom will lose, gain, or share electrons to fill its valence shell.

A neutral atom will have an equal number of protons and electrons. When a neutral atom loses or gains electrons, it gains or loses charge accordingly, forming an **ion**. An ion with more protons than electrons has a positive charge and is called a **cation**. An ion with more electrons than protons has a negative charge and is considered an **anion**.

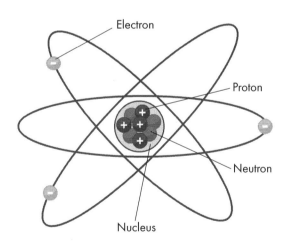

Figure 6.1. Structure of the Atom

 Helpful Hint: The attractive and repulsive forces in an atom follow the universal law that "like charges repel and opposite charges attract."

For example, the element oxygen (O) has eight protons and eight electrons. A neutral oxygen atom is represented simply as O. However, if it gains two electrons, it becomes an anion with a charge of −2 and is written as O^{2-}.

All atoms with the same number of protons are the same **element** and cannot be further reduced to a simpler substance by chemical processes. Each element has a symbol, which is a one- or two-letter abbreviation for the element's name. The number of protons in an atom is that atom's **atomic number**.

 Did You Know? Many element symbols are derived from the Latin names for elements. For example, the Latin name for *gold* is *aurum*, and its symbol is Au.

Along with atomic charge, atoms have measurable mass. Protons and neutrons are significantly more massive than electrons (about 1,800 times), so the mass of electrons is not considered when calculating the mass of an atom. Thus, an element's **mass number** is the number of protons and neutrons present in its atoms.

PRACTICE QUESTIONS

1. An atom with five protons and seven electrons has a charge of

    a.   −12

    b.   −2

    c.   2

    d.   5

    e.   12

Answer:

b. is correct. The total charge of an atom is the difference between the number of protons and electrons. Subtract the number of electrons from the number of protons: 5 − 7 = −2.

2. The ion with the greatest number of electrons is

    a. K^+

    b. Cl^-

    c. Ca^+

    d. P^{3-}

    e. S^{2-}

Answer:

c. is correct. Calcium has an atomic number of 20 (found on the periodic table), meaning it has twenty protons. For a Ca ion to have a charge of 1+, it must have nineteen electrons. All the other ions have eighteen electrons.

The Periodic Table of the Elements

Legend box:
Atomic Number
Symbol
Name
Atomic Mass

1	2	3	4	5	6	7	8	9	10	11	12	13	14	15	16	17	18
1 H Hydrogen 1.008																	2 He Helium 4.0026
3 Li Lithium 6.941	4 Be Beryllium 9.0122											5 B Boron 10.81	6 C Carbon 12.011	7 N Nitrogen 14.007	8 O Oxygen 15.999	9 F Fluorine 18.998	10 Ne Neon 20.180
11 Na Sodium 22.990	12 Mg Magnesium 24.305											13 Al Aluminum 26.982	14 Si Silicon 28.085	15 P Phosphorus 30.974	16 S Sulfur 32.06	17 Cl Chlorine 35.45	18 Ar Argon 39.948
19 K Potassium 39.098	20 Ca Calcium 40.078	21 Sc Scandium 44.956	22 Ti Titanium 47.867	23 V Vanadium 50.942	24 Cr Chromium 51.996	25 Mn Manganese 54.938	26 Fe Iron 55.845	27 Co Cobalt 58.933	28 Ni Nickel 58.963	29 Cu Copper 63.546	30 Zn Zinc 65.38	31 Ga Gallium 69.723	32 Ge Germanium 72.64	33 Es Arsenic 74.922	34 Se Selenium 78.971	35 Br Bromine 79.904	36 Kr Krypton 83.798
37 Rb Rubidium 85.468	38 Sr Strontium 87.62	39 Y Yttrium 88.906	40 Zr Zirconium 91.224	41 Nb Niobium 92.906	42 Mo Molybdenum 254	43 Tc Technetium 98	44 Ru Ruthenium 101.07	45 Rh Rhodium 102.91	46 Pd Palladium 106.42	47 Ag Silver 107.87	48 Cd Cadmium 112.41	49 In Indium 114.82	50 Sn Tin 118.71	51 Sb Antimony 121.76	52 Te Tellurium 127.60	53 I Iodine 126.90	54 Xe Xenon 121.29
55 Cs Caesium 132.91	56 Ba Barium 137.33	57-71	72 Hf Hafnium 178.49	73 Ta Tantalum 183.84	74 W Tungsten 183.84	75 Re Rhenium 186.21	76 Os Osmium 190.23	77 Ir Iridium 192.22	78 Pt Platinum 195.08	79 Au Gold 196.97	80 Hg Mercury 200.59	81 Tl Thallium 204.38	82 Pb Lead 207.2	83 Bi Bismuth 208.98	84 Po Polonium 209	85 At Astatine 210	86 Rn Radon 222
87 Fr Francium 223.020	88 Ra Radium 226	89-103	104 Rf Rutherfordium 267	105 Db Dubnium 268	106 Sg Seaborgium 271	107 Bh Bohrium 272	108 Hs Hassium 277	109 Mt Meitnerium 276	110 Ds Darmstadtium 281	111 Rg Roentgenium 280	112 Cn Copernicium 285	113 Uut Ununtrium Unknown	114 Fl Flerovium 254	115 Uup Ununpentium Unknown	116 Lv Livermorium 291	117 Uus Ununseptium Unknown	118 Uuo Ununoctium Unknown

Lanthanide

| 57 La Lanthanium 138.905 | 58 Ce Cerium 140.12 | 59 Pr Praseodymium 140.91 | 60 Nd Neodymium 144.24 | 61 Pm Promethium 144.913 | 62 Sm Samarium 150.36 | 63 Eu Europium 151.96 | 64 Gd Gadolinium 157.25 | 65 Tb Terbium 158.93 | 66 Dy Dysprosium 152.50 | 67 Ho Holmium 154.930 | 68 Er Erbium 167.259 | 69 Tm Thulium 168.934 | 70 Yb Ytterbium 173.065 | 71 Lu Lutetium 174.967 |

Actinide

| 89 Ac Actinium 227.028 | 90 Th Thorium 232.038 | 91 Pa Protactinium 231.036 | 92 U Uranium 238.029 | 93 Np Neptunium 237.048 | 94 Pu Plutonium 244.064 | 95 Am Americium 243.061 | 96 Cm Curium 247.070 | 97 Bk Berkelium 247.070 | 98 Cf Californium 251.080 | 99 Es Einsteinium 254 | 100 Fm Fermium 257.095 | 101 Md Mendelevium 258.1 | 102 No Nobelium 259.101 | 103 Lr Lawrencium 262 |

Legend:
- Alkaline Metal
- Alkaline Earth Metals
- Transition Metal
- Basic Metal
- Metalloid
- Nonmetal
- Halogen
- Noble Gas
- Lanthanide
- Actinide

Figure 6.2. The Periodic Table of the Elements

The Periodic Table of the Elements

Elements are arranged on the **Periodic Table of the Elements** by their atomic number, which increases from top to bottom and left to right on the table. Hydrogen, the first element on the periodic table, has one proton while helium, the second element, has two, and so on.

The rows of the periodic table are called **periods**, and the vertical columns are called **groups**. Each group contains elements with the same number of valence electrons, meaning the elements have similar chemical properties.

The majority of the elements in the periodic table are metals. Metals have the following properties:

+ They are hard, opaque, and shiny.
+ They are ductile and malleable.
+ They conduct electricity and heat.
+ With the exception of mercury, they are solids.

Metals begin on the left side of the periodic table and span across the middle of the table, almost all the way to the right side. Examples of metals include gold (Au), tin (Sn), and lead (Pb).

Nonmetals are elements that do not conduct electricity and tend to be more reactive than metals. They can be solids, liquids, or gases. The nonmetals are located on the right side of the periodic table. Examples of nonmetals include sulfur (S), hydrogen (H), and oxygen (O).

Metalloids, or semimetals, are elements that possess both metal and nonmetal characteristics. For example, some metalloids are shiny but do not conduct electricity well. Metalloids are located between the metals and nonmetals on the periodic table. Some examples of metalloids are boron (B), silicon (Si), and arsenic (As).

PRACTICE QUESTIONS

3. Bismuth is a
    a. metal
    b. nonmetal
    c. metalloid
    d. transition element
    e. noble gas

    Answer:

    a. is correct. Bismuth is a metal.

4. Fluorine is most likely to form an ionic compound with
    a. nickel (Ni)
    b. beryllium (Be)
    c. sodium (Na)
    d. argon (Ar)
    e. chlorine (Cl)

Chemical Bonds

Chemical bonds are attractions between atoms that create molecules, which are substances consisting of more than one atom. There are three types of bonds: ionic, covalent, and metallic.

In an **ionic bond**, one atom "gives" its electrons to the other, resulting in one positively and one negatively charged atom. The bond is a result of the attraction between the two ions. Ionic bonds form between atoms on the left side of the periodic table (which will lose electrons) and those on the right side (which will gain electrons). Table salt (NaCl) is an example of a molecule held together by an ionic bond.

A **covalent bond** is created by a pair of atoms sharing electrons to fill their valence shells. In a **nonpolar** covalent bond, the electrons are shared evenly. In a **polar** covalent bond, the electrons are shared unevenly. One atom will exert a stronger pull on the shared electrons, giving that atom a slight negative charge. The other atom in the bond will have a slight positive charge. Water (H_2O) is an example of a polar molecule.

Metals can form tightly packed arrays in which each atom is in close contact with many neighbors. The valence electrons are free to move between atoms and create a "sea" of delocalized charge. Any excitation, such as an electrical current, can cause the electrons to move throughout the array. The high electrical and thermal conductivity of metals is due to this ability of electrons to move throughout the lattice. This type of delocalized bonding is called **metallic bonding**.

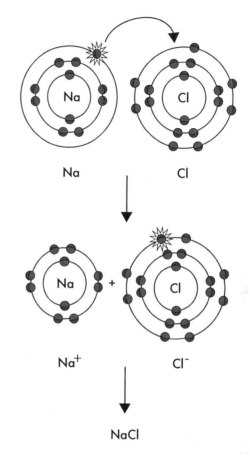

Na   Cl

Na⁺   Cl⁻

NaCl

Figure 6.3. The Ionic Bond in Table Salt

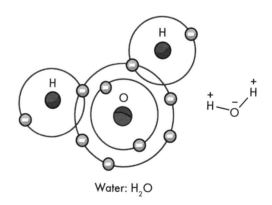

Water: H_2O

Figure 6.4. Polar Covalent Bond

Did You Know? The polar nature of water is responsible for many of its unique properties. The small charges within a water molecule cause attraction between the molecules. The molecules then "stick" to each other (cohesion) and to other surfaces (adhesion).

PRACTICE QUESTION

5. A polar covalent bond joins the atoms in the molecule

   a. LiF
   b. CO_2
   c. H_2
   d. NaOH
   e. O_2

   <u>Answer:</u>

   b. is correct. Carbon and oxygen are both nonmetals that combine through a covalent bond. Oxygen has a strong pull on their shared electrons, so CO_2 is polar. In hydrogen and oxygen gases, the identical atoms share electrons equally, so both compounds are nonpolar. Choices a and d are ionic compounds.

Properties of Matter

Matter is any substance that takes up space. The amount of matter in an object is that object's **mass**, which is measured in grams or kilograms. Mass is different from **weight**, which is a measure of the gravitational force exerted on an object. An object's mass never changes, but its weight will change if the gravitational force changes. The **density** of an object is the ratio of an object's mass to its volume.

> Did You Know? Objects weigh less on the moon than on the earth because the pull of gravity on the moon is lower than that on earth. However, the mass of the object is the same no matter where in the universe it goes.

Properties of substances are divided into two categories: physical and chemical. **Physical properties** are those that are measurable and can be seen without changing the chemical makeup of a substance. In contrast, **chemical properties** are those that determine how a substance will behave in a chemical reaction. Chemical properties cannot be identified simply by observing a material. Instead, the material must be engaged in a chemical reaction in order to identify its chemical properties. A **physical change** is a change in a substance's physical properties, and a **chemical change** is a change in its chemical properties.

Table 6.1. Properties of Matter

Physical Properties	Chemical Properties
mass	heat of combustion
temperature	flammability
density	toxicity
color	chemical stability
viscosity	enthalpy of formation

Temperature is the name given to the kinetic energy of all the atoms or molecules in a substance. While it might look like matter is not in motion, in fact, its atoms have kinetic energy and are constantly spinning and vibrating. The more energy the atoms have (meaning the more they spin and vibrate) the higher the substance's temperature.

Heat is the movement of energy from one substance to another. Energy will spontaneously move from high-energy (high-temperature) substances to low-energy (low-temperature) substances.

PRACTICE QUESTION

6.   A substance that can change shape but not volume is a

   a.   solid

   b.   liquid

   c.   gas

   d.   solid or liquid

   e.   liquid or gas

   Answer:

   b. is correct. Liquids can change shape (for instance, when they are poured from one container into another) but not volume.

States of Matter

All matter exists in different **states** (or phases) that depend on the energy of the molecules in the matter. **Solid** matter has densely packed molecules and does not change volume or shape. **Liquids** have more loosely packed molecules and can change shape but not volume. **Gas** molecules are widely dispersed, and gases can change both shape and volume.

Changes in temperature and pressure can cause matter to change states. Generally, adding energy (in the form of heat) changes a substance to a higher energy state (e.g., solid to liquid). Transitions from a high to lower energy state (e.g., liquid to solid) release energy. Each of these changes has a specific name, summarized in the table below.

Table 6.2. Changes in State of Matter

Name	From	To	Occurs At	Enery Change
evaporation	liquid	gas	boiling point	uses energy
condensation	gas	liquid	boiling point	releases energy
melting	solid	liquid	freezing point	uses energy
freezing	liquid	solid	freezing point	releases energy

Name	From	To	Occurs At	Enery Change
sublimation	solid	gas	---	uses energy
deposition	gas	solid	---	releases energy

Table 6.2. Changes in State of Matter (continued)

PRACTICE QUESTION

7. The process that takes place when water reaches its boiling point is called
    a. condensation
    b. evaporation
    c. melting
    d. sublimation
    e. freezing

    Answer:

    b. is correct. Evaporation is the process of conversion from liquid to gas that occurs at the boiling point.

Chemical Reactions

A **chemical reaction** occurs when one or more substances react to form new substances. **Reactants** are the substances that are consumed or altered in the chemical reaction, and the new substances are **products**. Equations are written with the reactants on the left, the products on the right, and an arrow between them. The state of the chemical compounds are sometimes noted using the labels s (solid), l (liquid), g (gas), or aq (aqueous, meaning a solution).

The equation below shows the reaction of hydrogen gas (H_2) and chlorine gas (Cl_2) to form hydrogen chloride (HCl), an acid.

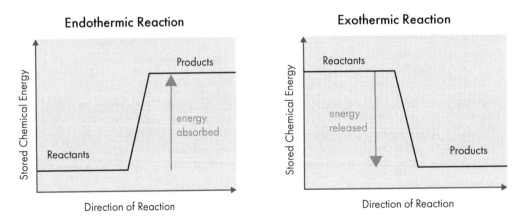

Figure 6.5. Stored Energy in Endothermic and Exothermic Reactions

$$H_2 \ (g) + Cl_2 \ (g) \rightarrow 2HCl \ (aq)$$

Chemical reactions follow the **law of conservation of matter**, which states that matter cannot be created or destroyed. In a reaction, the same types and numbers of atoms that appear on the left side must also appear on the right. To **balance** a chemical equation, coefficients (the numbers before the reactant or product) are added. In the equation above, a coefficient of two is needed on HCl so that two hydrogen and two chlorine atoms appear on each side of the arrow.

There are five main types of chemical reactions; these are summarized in the table below.

Table 6.3. Types of Reactions

Type of Reaction	General Formula	Example Reaction
Synthesis	$A + B \rightarrow C$	$2H_2 + O_2 \rightarrow 2H_2O$
Decomposition	$A \rightarrow B + C$	$2H_2O_2 \rightarrow 2H_2O + O_2$
Single displacement	$AB + C \rightarrow A + BC$	$CH_4 + Cl_2 \rightarrow CH_3Cl + HCl$
Double displacement	$AB + CD \rightarrow AC + BD$	$CuCl_2 + 2AgNo_3 \rightarrow Cu(NO_3)_2 + 2AgCl$
Combustion	$C_xH_y + O_2 \rightarrow CO_2 + H_2O$	$2C_8H_{18} + 25O_2 \rightarrow 16CO_2 + 18H_2O$

Energy is required to break chemical bonds, and it is released when bonds form. The total energy absorbed or released during a chemical reaction will depend on the individual bonds being broken and formed. A reaction that releases energy is **exothermic**, and a reaction that absorbs energy is **endothermic**.

PRACTICE QUESTIONS

8. $Pb(NO_3)_2 + K_2CrO_4 \rightarrow PbCrO_4 + 2KNO_3$

The reaction shown above is a

a.   combustion reaction

b.   decomposition reaction

c.   double-displacement reaction

d.   single-replacement reaction

e.   acid-base neutralization reaction

Answer:

c. is correct. In the reaction, Pb and K exchange their anions in a double-displacement reaction.

9.   An example of a balanced equation is

a. $KClO_3 \rightarrow KCl + 3O_2$

b. $2KClO_3 \rightarrow KCl + 2O_2$

c. $2KClO_3 \rightarrow 2KCl + 3O_2$

d. $4KClO_3 \rightarrow 2KCl + 2O_2$

e. $6KClO_3 \rightarrow 6KCl + 3O_2$

<u>Answer:</u>

c. is correct. In this equation, there are equal numbers of each type of atom on both sides (two K atoms, two Cl atoms, and six O atoms).

Mixtures

When substances are combined without a chemical reaction to bond them, the resulting substance is called a **mixture**. Physical changes can be used to separate mixtures. For example, heating salt water until the water evaporates, leaving the salt behind, will separate a salt water solution.

In a mixture, the components can be unevenly distributed, such as in trail mix or soil. These mixtures are described at **heterogeneous**. Alternatively, the components can be **homogeneously**, or uniformly, distributed, as in salt water.

A **solution** is a special type of stable homogeneous mixture. The components of a solution will not separate on their own and cannot be separated using a filter. The substance being dissolved is the **solute**, and the substance acting on the solute, or doing the dissolving, is the **solvent**.

> Did You Know? Solutions can exist as solids, liquids, or gases. For example, carbonated water has a gaseous solute (CO_2) and a liquid solvent (water). A solution formed by combining two solid metals, such as stainless steel, is an **alloy**.

The **solubility** of a solution is the maximum amount of solute that will dissolve in a specific quantity of solvent at a specified temperature. Solutions can be saturated, unsaturated, or supersaturated based on the amount of solute dissolved in the solution.

✦ A **saturated** solution has the maximum amount of solute that can be dissolved in the solvent.

✦ An **unsaturated** solution contains less solute than a saturated solution would hold.

✦ A **supersaturated solution** contains more solvent than a saturated solution. A supersaturated solution can be made by heating the solution to dissolve additional solute and then slowly cooling it down to a specified temperature.

PRACTICE QUESTIONS

10. A heterogeneous mixture is one in which

    a. the atoms or molecules are distributed unevenly

    b. two substances are in different states

    c. there is a mixture of covalent and ionic compounds

    d. there is a mixture of polar and nonpolar molecules

    e. three or more different molecules are mixed together

Answer:

a. is correct. A heterogeneous mixture is any nonuniform mixture, which means the atoms or molecules are unevenly distributed.

11. A solution in which more solvent can be dissolved is called
    a. unsaturated
    b. saturated
    c. supersaturated
    d. homogeneous
    e. heterogeneous

Answer:

a. is correct. An unsaturated solution has less solute than can be dissolved in the given amount of solvent.

Acids and Bases

Acids and bases are substances that share a distinct set of physical properties. **Acids** are corrosive, sour, and change the color of vegetable dyes like litmus from blue to red. **Bases**, or alkaline solutions, are slippery, bitter, and change the color of litmus from red to blue.

There are a number of different ways to define acids and bases, but generally acids release hydrogen ions (H^+) in solution, while bases release hydroxide (OH^-) ions. For example, hydrochloric acid (HCl) ionizes, or breaks apart, in solution to release H^+ ions:

$$HCl \rightarrow H^+ + Cl$$

The base sodium hydroxide (NaOH) ionizes to release OH^- ions:

$$NaOH \rightarrow Na^+ + OH^-$$

Acids and bases combine in a **neutralization reaction**. During the reaction, the H^+ and OH^- ions join to form water, and the remaining ions combine to form a salt:

$$HCl + NaOH \rightarrow H_2O + NaCl$$

Did You Know? A **buffer**, or buffer solution, is a solution that resists changes in pH when small quantities of acids or bases are added. A buffer can do this because it contains a weak acid to react with any added base and a weak base to react with any added acid.

The strength of an acid or base is measured on the **pH scale**, which ranges from 1 to 14, with 1 being the strongest acid, 14 being the strongest base, and 7 being neutral. A substance's pH value is a measure of how many hydrogen ions are in the solution. The scale is logarithmic, meaning an acid with a pH of 3 has ten times as many hydrogen ions as an acid with a pH of 4. Water, which separates into equal numbers of H^+ and OH^- ions, has a neutral pH of 7.

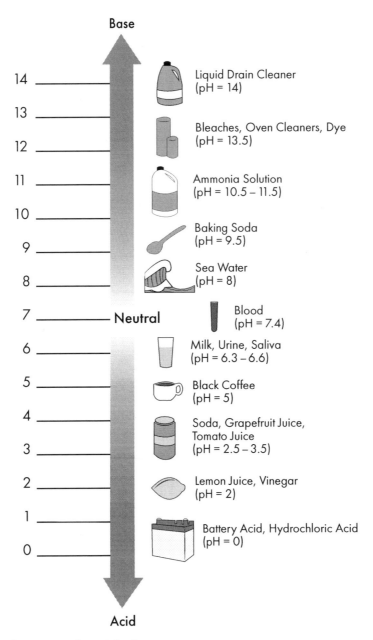

Base

14 —————— Liquid Drain Cleaner
 (pH = 14)

13 ——————

12 —————— Bleaches, Oven Cleaners, Dye
 (pH = 13.5)

11 —————— Ammonia Solution
 (pH = 10.5 – 11.5)

10 ——————

9 —————— Baking Soda
 (pH = 9.5)

8 —————— Sea Water
 (pH = 8)

7 —————— Neutral   Blood
 (pH = 7.4)

6 —————— Milk, Urine, Saliva
 (pH = 6.3 – 6.6)

5 —————— Black Coffee
 (pH = 5)

4 —————— Soda, Grapefruit Juice,
 Tomato Juice
3 —————— (pH = 2.5 – 3.5)

2 —————— Lemon Juice, Vinegar
 (pH = 2)

1 —————— Battery Acid, Hydrochloric Acid
 (pH = 0)
0 ——————

Acid

Figure 6.6. The pH Scale

PRACTICE QUESTIONS

12. A neutralization reaction produces

  a. a base

  b. a buffer

  c. hydrogen ions

  d. a salt

  e. an acid

Answer:

d. is correct. A neutralization reaction occurs when an acid and a base combine to form a salt and water.

13. When a nitric acid solution is diluted by a factor of ten, the pH will

    a. go up ten units

    b. go down ten units

    c. go up one unit

    d. go down one unit

    e. stay the same

Answer:

c. is correct. The pH will go up: diluting an acid will decrease the concentration of H^+ ions, and higher pH values represent lower concentrations of H^+ ions. Diluting the acid by a factor of ten will change the pH one unit because the pH scale is logarithmic.

Motion

To study motion, it is necessary to understand the concept of scalars and vectors. **Scalars** are measurements that have a quantity but no direction. **Vectors**, in contrast, have both a quantity and a direction. **Distance** is a scalar: it describes how far an object has traveled along a path. Distance can have values such as 54 m or 16 miles. **Displacement** is a vector: it describes how far an object has traveled from its starting position. A displacement value will indicate direction, such as 54 m east or −16 miles.

Table 6.4. Physical Science Units	
mass	kilograms (kg)
displacement	meters (m)
velocity	meters per second (m/s)
acceleration	meters per second per second (m/s^2)
force	Newtons (N)
work	Joules (J)
energy	Joules (J)
current	amperes (A)
voltage	volts (V)

Speed describes how quickly something is moving. It is found by dividing distance by time, and so is a scalar value. **Velocity** is the rate at which an object changes position. Velocity is found by dividing displacement by time, meaning it is a vector value. An object that travels a certain distance and then returns to its starting point has a velocity of zero because its final position did not change. Its speed, however, can be found by dividing the total distance it traveled by the time it took to make the trip.

Acceleration describes how quickly an object changes velocity. It is also a vector: when acceleration is in the same direction as velocity, the object will move faster. When the acceleration is in the opposite direction of velocity, the object will slow down.

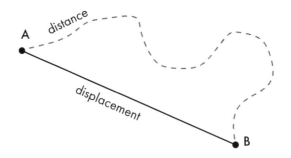

Figure 6.7. Distance versus Displacement

PRACTICE QUESTION

14. A person who starts from rest and increases his velocity to 5 m/s over a time period of 1 second has an acceleration of

   a.   −5 m/s²
   b.   0 m/s²
   c.   1 m/s²
   d.   5 m/s²
   e.   10 m/s²

   <u>Answer:</u>

   d. is correct. Acceleration is the change in velocity over the change in time:

   $a = \frac{v}{t} = \frac{(5 \text{ m/s} - 0 \text{ m/s})}{1 \text{ s}} = \textbf{5 m/s}^2$

Forces

A push or pull that causes an object to move or change direction is called a **force**. Forces can arise from a number of different sources.

   ✦   **Gravity** is the attraction of one mass to another mass. For example, the earth's gravitational field pulls objects toward it, and the sun's gravitational field keeps planets in motion around it.

   ✦   **Electrical force** is the creation of a field by charged particles that will cause other charged objects in that field to move.

   ✦   **Tension** is found in ropes pulling or holding up an object.

   ✦   **Friction** is created by two objects moving against each other.

   ✦   **Normal force** occurs when an object is resting on another object.

   ✦   **Buoyant force** is the upward force experienced by floating objects.

In 1687, Isaac Newton published **three laws of motion** that describe the behavior of force and mass. Newton's first law is also called the **law of inertia**. It states that an object will maintain its current state of motion unless acted on by an outside force.

Newton's **second law** is an equation, $F = ma$. The equation states that increasing the force on an object will increase its acceleration. In addition, the mass of the object will determine its acceleration: under the same force, a small object will accelerate more quickly than a larger object.

An object in equilibrium is either at rest or is moving at constant velocity; in other words, the object has no acceleration, or $a = 0$. Using Newton's second law, an object is in equilibrium if the net force on the object is 0, or $F = 0$ (this is called the equilibrium condition).

Newton's **third law** states that for every action (force), there will be an equal and opposite reaction (force). For instance, if a person is standing on the floor, there is a force of gravity pulling him toward the earth. However, he is not accelerating toward the earth; he is simply standing at rest on the floor (in equilibrium). So, the floor must provide a force that is equal in magnitude and in the opposite direction to the force of gravity.

PRACTICE QUESTIONS

15. A book resting on a table is prevented from falling on the floor by

a. gravity

b. tension

c. friction

d. electromagnetic force

e. normal force

Answer:

e. is correct. The normal force pushes up to counterbalance the force of gravity, which points down.

16. An example of an object in equilibrium is

a. a parachutist after he jumps from an airplane

b. an airplane taking off

c. a person sitting still in a chair

d. a soccer ball when it is kicked

e. the moon orbiting the earth

Answer:

c. is correct. A person sitting in a chair is not accelerating. All the other choices describe objects that are accelerating or changing velocity.

Work

Work is a scalar value that is defined as the application of a force over a distance. It is measured in Joules (J).

A person lifting a book off the ground is an example of someone doing work. The book has a weight because it is being pulled toward the earth. As the person lifts the book, her hand and arm are producing a force that is larger than that weight, causing the book to rise. The higher the person lifts the book, the more work is done.

The sign of the work done is important. In the example of lifting a book, the person's hand is doing positive (+) work on the book. However, gravity is always pulling the book down, which means that during a lift, gravity is doing negative (–) work on the book. If the force and the displacement are in the same direction, then the work is positive (+). If the force and the displacement are in opposite directions, then the work is negative (–). In the case of lifting a book, the net work done on the book is positive.

PRACTICE QUESTION

17.   The most work is done on a car when

   a.   pushing on the car, but it does not move

   b.   towing the car up a steep hill for 100 m

   c.   pushing the car 5 m across a parking lot

   d.   painting the car

   e.   driving the car in reverse for 5 m

   Answer:

   b. is correct. A steep hill requires a large force to counter the gravitational force. The large distance will also lead to a large amount of work done. Less work is done in choices c and e, and no work is done in choice a. Choice d is incorrect because painting the car is "work," but not the technical definition of work. The car is not moving while being painted, so no work is done on the car.

Energy

Energy is an abstract concept, but everything in nature has an energy associated with it. Energy is measured in Joules (J). There are many types of energy:

   + mechanical: the energy of motion

   + chemical: the energy in chemical bonds

   + thermal: the energy of an object due to its temperature

   + nuclear: the energy in the nucleus of an atom

   + electric: the energy arising from charged particles

   + magnetic: the energy arising from a magnetic field

There is an energy related to movement called the **kinetic energy (KE)**. Any object that has mass and is moving will have a kinetic energy.

Potential energy (PE) is the energy stored in a system; it can be understood as the potential for an object to gain kinetic energy. There are several types of potential energy.

+ **Electric potential energy** is derived from the interaction between positive and negative charges.

+ Compressing a spring stores **elastic potential energy**.

+ Energy is also stored in chemical bonds as **chemical potential energy**.

+ The energy stored by objects due to their height is **gravitational potential energy**.

Energy can be converted into other forms of energy, but it cannot be created or destroyed. This principle is called the **conservation of energy**. A swing provides a simple example of this principle. Throughout the swing's path, the total energy of the system remains the same. At the highest point of a swing's path, it has potential energy but no kinetic energy (because it has stopped moving momentarily as it changes direction). As the swing drops, that potential energy is converted to kinetic energy, and the swing's velocity increases. At the bottom of its path, all its potential energy has been converted into kinetic energy (meaning its potential energy is zero). This process repeats as the swing moves up and down. At any point in the swing's path, the kinetic and potential energies will sum to the same value.

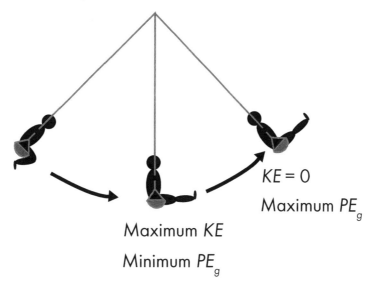

Figure 6.8. Conservation of Energy in a Swing

PRACTICE QUESTION

18. The energy stored in a compressed spring is

    a. nuclear energy

    b. mechanical energy

    c. chemical potential energy

    d. gravitational potential energy

    e. elastic potential energy

Waves

Energy can also be transferred through **waves**, which are repeating pulses of energy. Waves that travel through a medium, like ripples on a pond or compressions in a Slinky, are called **mechanical waves**. Waves that vibrate up and down (like the ripples on a pond) are **transverse waves**, and those that travel through compression (like the Slinky) are **longitudinal waves**. Mechanical waves will travel faster through denser mediums; for example, sound waves will move faster through water than through air.

Waves can be described using a number of different properties. A wave's highest point is called its **crest**, and its lowest point is the **trough**. A wave's **midline** is halfway between the crest and trough; the **amplitude** describes the distance between the midline and the crest (or trough). The distance between crests (or troughs) is the **wavelength**. A wave's **period** is the time it takes for a wave to go through one complete cycle, and the number of cycles a wave goes through in a specific period of time is its **frequency**.

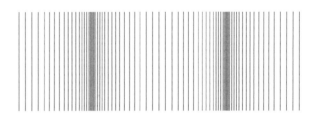

Longitudinal Wave

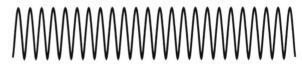

Transverse Wave

Figure 6.9. Types of Waves

Sound is a special type of longitudinal wave created by vibrations. Our ears are able to interpret these waves as particular sounds. The frequency, or rate, of the vibration determines the sound's **pitch**. **Loudness** depends on the amplitude, or height, of a sound wave.

The **Doppler effect** is the difference in perceived pitch caused by the motion of the object creating the wave. For example, as an ambulance approaches an observer, the siren's pitch will appear to increase, and then as the ambulance moves away, the siren's pitch will appear to decrease. This occurs because sound waves are compressed as the ambulance approaches the observer and are spread out as the ambulance moves away from the observer.

Electromagnetic waves are composed of oscillating electric and magnetic fields and thus do not require a medium through which to travel. The electromagnetic spectrum classifies the types of electromagnetic waves based on their frequency. These include radio waves, microwaves, X-rays, and visible light.

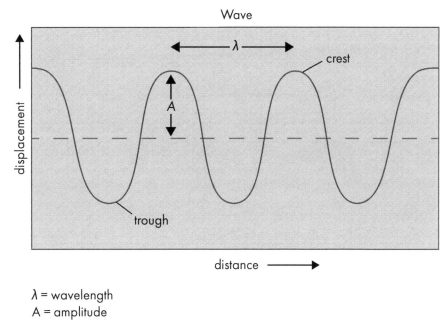

λ = wavelength
A = amplitude

Figure 6.10. Parts of a Wave

The study of light is called **optics**. Because visible light is a wave, it will display properties that are similar to other waves. It will **reflect**, or bounce off, surfaces, which can be observed by shining a flashlight on a mirror. Light will also **refract**, or bend, when it travels between substances. This effect can be seen by placing a pencil in water and observing the apparent bend in the pencil.

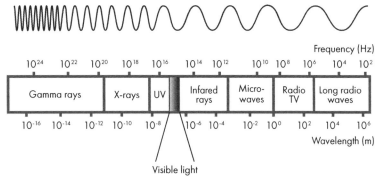

Figure 6.11. The Electromagnetic Spectrum

Curved pieces of glass called **lenses** can be used to bend light in a way that affects how an image is perceived. Some microscopes, for example, make objects appear larger through the use of specific types of lenses. Eyeglasses also use lenses to correct poor vision.

The frequency of a light wave is responsible for its color, with red/orange colors having a lower frequency than blue/violet colors. White light is a blend of all the frequencies of visible light. Passing white light through a prism will bend each frequency at a slightly different angle, separating the colors and creating a rainbow. Sunlight passing through raindrops can undergo this effect, creating large rainbows in the sky.

19. Refraction, the bending of waves, can cause

    a.   rainbows

    b.   echoes

    c.   loudness

    d.   reflections in mirrors

    e.   the Doppler effect

<u>Answer:</u>

a. is correct. Rainbows are created when light passes through an object, such as a raindrop or prism, that causes the colors in light to bend at different angles.

Electricity and Magnetism

Electric charge is created by a difference in the balance of protons and electrons, which creates a positively or negatively charged object. Charged objects create an **electric field** that spreads outward from the object. Other charged objects in that field will experience a force: objects that have opposite charges will be attracted to each other, and objects with the same charge will be repelled, or pushed away, from each other.

Because protons cannot leave the nucleus, charge is created by the movement of electrons. **Static electricity**, or electrostatic charge, occurs when a surface has a buildup of charges. For example, if a student rubs a balloon on her head, the friction will cause electrons to move from her hair to the balloon. This creates a negative charge on the balloon and a positive charge on her hair; the resulting attraction will cause her hair to move toward the balloon.

Electricity is the movement of electrons through a conductor, and an electric circuit is a closed loop through which electricity moves. Circuits include a **voltage** source, which powers the movement of electrons known as **current**. Sources of voltage include batteries, generators, and wall outlets (which are in turn powered by electric power stations). Other elements, such as lights, computers, and microwaves, can then be connected to the circuit and then powered by its electricity.

Magnets are created by the alignment of spinning electrons within a substance. This alignment will occur naturally in some substances, including iron, nickel, and cobalt, all of which can be used to produce permanent magnets. The alignment of electrons creates a magnetic field, which, like an electric or gravitational field, can act on other objects. Magnetic fields have a north and a south pole that act similarly to electric charges: opposite poles will attract, and same poles will repel each other. However, unlike electric charge, which can be either positive or negative, a magnetic field ALWAYS has two poles. If a magnet is cut in half, the result is two magnets, each with a north and a south pole.

Electricity and magnetism are closely related. A moving magnet creates an electric field, and a moving charged particle creates a magnetic field. A specific kind of temporary magnet known as an **electromagnet** can be made by coiling a wire around a metal object and running electricity through it. A magnetic field will be created when the wire contains a current but will disappear when the flow of electricity is stopped.

PRACTICE QUESTION

20. The particles that flow through a circuit to power a light bulb are

    a.   protons

    b.   neutrons

    c.   electrons

    d.   nucleus

    e.   atoms

Answer:

c. is correct. Electrons are negatively charged subatomic particles that exist outside the nucleus of an atom. A power source forces moving electrons through a circuit.

Test Your Knowledge

Read the question, and then choose the most correct answer.

1. Which of the following determines the atomic number of an atom?

    a. the number of electrons orbiting the nucleus

    b. the number of protons in the nucleus

    c. the number of protons and neutrons in the nucleus

    d. the number of protons and electrons in the atom

2. How many neutrons are in an atom of the element $^{88}_{38}$Sr?

    a. 38

    b. 88

    c. 50

    d. 126

3. Refer to the periodic table in Figure 6.2. Which element is a metalloid?

    a. rubidium

    b. vanadium

    c. antimony

    d. iodine

4. Which of the following is NOT a typical property of metals?

    a. Metals have low densities.

    b. Metals are malleable.

    c. Metals are good conductors of electricity and heat.

    d. Metals in solid state consist of ordered structures with tightly packed atoms.

5. Which element has chemical properties most similar to sulfur?

    a. fluorine

    b. argon

    c. phosphorus

    d. oxygen

6. Which of the following groups on the periodic table will typically adopt a charge of +1 when forming ionic compounds?

    a. alkaline earth metals

    b. lanthanides

    c. actinides

    d. alkali metals

7. Match the elements with the type of bond that would occur between them.

Elements	Bond
magnesium and bromine	
carbon and oxygen	
solid copper	

    a. ionic

    b. metallic

    c. covalent

8. Label each compound as polar or nonpolar.

Compound	Polar	Nonpolar
H_2O		
F_2		
HF		

9. How many electrons are included in the double bond between the two oxygen atoms in O_2?

   a. 2
   b. 4
   c. 6
   d. 8

10. Which of the following describes a physical change?

    a. Water becomes ice.
    b. Batter is baked into a cake.
    c. An iron fence rusts.
    d. A firecracker explodes.

11. Which of the following processes produces a gas from a solid?

    a. melting
    b. evaporation
    c. condensation
    d. sublimation

12. Which of the following is a double-replacement reaction?

    a. HNO_3 (aq) + NaOH (aq) → $NaNO_3$ (aq) + H_2O (l)
    b. CS_2 (g) + CO_2 (g) → 2COS (g)
    c. $2N_2O$ (g) → $2N_2$ (g) + O_2 (g)
    d. $BaCl_2$ (aq) + H_2SO_4 (aq) → 2HCl (aq) + $BaSO_4$ (s)

13. Balance the following chemical equation:

    $P_4 + O_2 + H_2O → H_3PO_4$

    a. 1:8:6:4
    b. 1:2:2:4
    c. 1:2:6:4
    d. 1:5:6:4

14. Which of the following is NOT a homogeneous mixture?

    a. air
    b. sandy water
    c. brass
    d. salt dissolved in water

15. Which trait defines a saturated solution?

    a. Both the solute and solvent are liquid.
    b. The solute is distributed evenly throughout the solution.
    c. The solute is unevenly distributed throughout the solution.
    d. No more solute can be dissolved in the solution.

16. Which of the following is NOT a definition of an acid?

    a. A substance that contains hydrogen and produces H^+ in water.
    b. A substance that donates protons to a base.
    c. A substance that reacts with a base to form a salt and water.
    d. A substance that accepts protons.

17. A ball is tossed straight into the air with a velocity of 3 m/s. What will its velocity be at its maximum height?

    a. −3 m/s
    b. 0 m/s
    c. 1.5 m/s
    d. 3 m/s

18. How far will a car moving at 40 m/s travel in 2 seconds?

    a. 10 m
    b. 20 m
    c. 40 m
    d. 80 m

19. If a baseball thrown straight up in the air takes 5 seconds to reach its peak, how long will it need to fall back to the player's hand?

    a.   2.5 seconds

    b.   9.8 seconds

    c.   5.0 seconds

    d.   10.0 seconds

20. Which of the following is a measure of the inertia of an object?

    a.   mass

    b.   speed

    c.   acceleration

    d.   force

21. A box sliding down a ramp experiences all of the following forces EXCEPT

    a.   tension.

    b.   friction.

    c.   gravitational.

    d.   normal.

22. A person with a mass of 80 kg travels to the moon, where the acceleration due to gravity is 1.62 m/s^2. What will her mass be on the moon?

    a.   greater than 80 kg

    b.   80 kg

    c.   less than 80 kg

    d.   The answer cannot be determined without more information.

23. If a force of 300 N is pushing on a block to the right and a force of 400 N is pushing on a block to the left, what is the net force on the block?

    a.   0 N

    b.   100 N to the left

    c.   300 N to the right

    d.   400 N to the left

24. A man is pushing against a heavy rock sitting on a flat plane, and the rock is not moving. The force that holds the rock in place is

    a.   friction.

    b.   gravity.

    c.   normal force.

    d.   buoyant force.

25. Which of the following describes what will happen when positive work is done on an object?

    a.   The object will gain energy.

    b.   The object will lose energy.

    c.   The object will increase its temperature.

    d.   The object will decrease its temperature.

26. What type of energy is stored in the bond between hydrogen and oxygen in water (H_2O)?

    a.   mechanical

    b.   chemical

    c.   nuclear

    d.   electric

27. A microscope makes use of which property of waves to make objects appear larger?

    a.   diffraction

    b.   amplitude

    c.   reflection

    d.   refraction

28. Which measurement describes the distance between crests in a wave?

    a.   amplitude

    b.   wavelength

    c.   frequency

    d.   period

29. Two negative charges are being held 1 meter apart. What will the charges do when they are released?

    a.   They will move closer together.

    b.   They will move farther apart.

    c.   They will stay 1 meter apart and move in the same direction.

    d.   They will stay 1 meter apart and not move.

30. The north poles of two magnets are held near each other. At which distance will the magnets experience the most force?

    a.   0.1 meters

    b.   1 meters

    c.   10 meters

    d.   100 meters

ANSWER KEY

1. **b.**

Atomic number is defined as the total number of protons in the nucleus of an atom.

2. **c.**

Subtracting the atomic number from the mass number gives the number of protons: $A - Z = 88 - 38 = 50$.

3. **c.**

Antimony is a metalloid. Rubidium is a metal, vanadium is a transition metal, and iodine is a halogen.

4. **a.**

Because metals tend to consist of ordered, tightly packed atoms, their densities are typically high (not low).

5. **d.**

Oxygen is in the same group as sulfur and is also a nonmetal.

6. **d.**

By losing one electron and thereby adopting a +1 charge, alkali metals achieve a noble gas electron configuration, making them more stable.

7.

Elements	Bond
magnesium and bromine	**a. is correct.** Ionic bonds form between elements on the left side of the periodic table and the right side.
carbon and oxygen	**c. is correct.** Nonmetals tend to form covalent bonds.
solid copper	**b. is correct.** Solid metals are held together by metallic bonding.

8.

Compound	Polar	Nonpolar
H_2O	O attracts electrons more strongly than H, and H_2O is bent such that the charges on each O do not balance.	
F_2		Because the two atoms are the same, they share electrons equally.
HF	F attracts electrons more strongly than H, creating a polar molecule.	

9. **b.**

The two oxygen atoms in a covalent double bond share two pairs of electrons, or four total.

10. **a.**

When water changes form, it does not change the chemical composition of the substance. Once water becomes ice, the ice can easily turn back into water.

11. **d.**

Sublimation is the phase change in which a material moves directly from the solid phase to the gas phase, bypassing the liquid phase.

12. **d.**

This reaction is a double-replacement reaction in which the two reactants change partners. Ba^{+2} combines with SO_4^{-2} and H^{+1} combines with Cl^{-1}.

13. **d.**

$\_P_4 + \_O_2 + \_H_2O \rightarrow \_H_3PO_4$
Add a 4 on the right side to balance the four P atoms on the left.

$\_P_4 + \_O_2 + \_H_2O \rightarrow 4H_3PO_4$
There are now twelve H atoms on the right, so add a 6 to H_2O on the left.

$\_P_4 + \_O_2 + 6H_2O \rightarrow 4H_3PO_4$
There are sixteen O on the right, so add a 5 to O_2 on the left.

$P_4 + 5O_2 + 6H_2O \rightarrow 4H_3PO_4$

14. **b.**

Sandy water is not a homogeneous mixture. Sand and water can be easily separated, making it a heterogeneous mixture.

15. **d.**

No more solute can be dissolved into a saturated solution.

16. **d.**

Acids increase the concentration of hydrogen ions in solution and do not accept protons.

17. **b.**

The velocity of a projectile is zero at its maximum height.

18. **d.**

Displacement is equal to velocity multiplied by time:
$d = vt = (40 \text{ m/s})(2 \text{ s}) = 80 \text{ m}$

19. **c.**

The time to the peak and the time to fall back to the original height are equal.

20. **a.**

Mass is a measure of an object's inertia.

21. **a.**

Tension is the force that results from objects being pulled or hung.

22. **b.**

The mass of an object is constant, so the mass would still be 80 kg. (However, the person's weight would be lower on the moon than on the earth.)

23. **b.**

The total force on an object is found by adding all the individual forces: 300 N + (−400 N) = −100 N (where negative is to the left).

24. **a.**

When the man pushes on the rock, static friction points opposite the direction of the applied force with the same magnitude. The forces add to zero, so the rock's acceleration is also zero.

25. a.

The object will gain energy.

26. b.

Chemical energy is stored in the bonds between atoms.

27. d.

Lenses refract, or bend, light waves to make objects appear larger.

28. b.

Wavelength is the length of each cycle of the wave, which can be found by measuring between crests.

29. b.

Like charges repel each other, so the two charges will move apart from each other.

30. a.

Magnetic force is inversely proportional to the distance between two objects, so the smallest distance will create the largest force.

SEVEN: EARTH AND SPACE SCIENCE

Astronomy

Astronomy is the study of space. Our planet, **Earth**, is just one out of a group of planets that orbit the sun, which is the star at the center of our solar system. Other planets in our solar system include Mercury, Venus, Mars, Jupiter, Saturn, Uranus, and Neptune. Every planet, except Mercury and Venus, has **moons**, or naturally occurring satellites that orbit a planet. Our solar system also includes **asteroids** and **comets**, small rocky or icy objects that orbit the Sun. Many of these are clustered in the **asteroid belt**, which is located between the orbits of Mars and Jupiter.

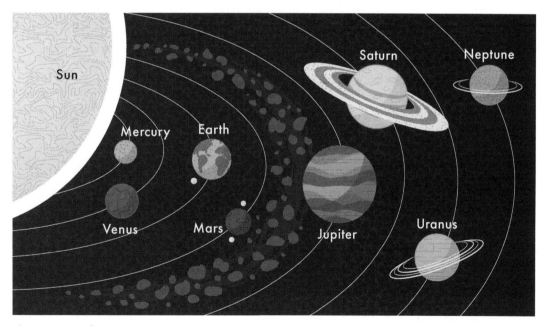

Figure 7.1. Solar System

Our solar system is a small part of a bigger star system called a **galaxy**. (Our galaxy is called the Milky Way.) Galaxies consist of stars, gas, and dust held together by gravity and contain millions of **stars**, which are hot balls of plasma and gases. The universe includes many types of stars, including supergiant stars, white dwarfs, giant stars, and neutron stars. Stars form in **nebulas**, which are large clouds of dust and gas. When very large stars collapse, they create **black holes**, which have a gravitational force so strong that light cannot escape.

Earth, the moon, and the sun interact in a number of ways that impact life on our planet. When the positions of the three align, eclipses occur. A **lunar eclipse** occurs when Earth lines up between the moon and the sun; the moon moves into the shadow of Earth and appears dark in color. A **solar eclipse** occurs when the moon lines up between Earth and the sun; the moon covers the sun, blocking sunlight.

The cycle of day and night and the seasonal cycle are determined by the earth's motion. It takes approximately 365 days, or one **year**, for Earth to revolve around the sun. While Earth is revolving around the sun, it is also rotating on its axis, which takes approximately twenty-four hours, or one **day**. As the planet rotates, different areas alternately face toward the sun and away from the sun, creating night and day.

The earth's axis is not directly perpendicular to its orbit, meaning the planet tilts on its axis. The **seasons** are caused by this tilt. When the Northern Hemisphere is tilted toward the sun, it receives more sunlight and experiences summer. At the same time that the Northern Hemisphere experiences summer, the Southern Hemisphere, which receives less direct sunlight, experiences winter. As the earth revolves, the Northern Hemisphere will tilt away from the sun and move into winter, while the Southern Hemisphere tilts toward the sun and moves into summer.

PRACTICE QUESTION

1. The phenomenon that occurs when the moon moves between the earth and the sun is called a(n)

    a. aurora
    b. lunar eclipse
    c. black hole
    d. solar eclipse
    e. solstice

    Answer:
    d. is correct. When the moon moves between the earth and the sun, a solar eclipse occurs, blocking sunlight from the planet.

Geology

Geology is the study of the minerals and rocks that make up the earth. A **mineral** is a naturally occurring, solid, inorganic substance with a crystalline structure. There are several properties that help identify a mineral, including color, luster, hardness, and density. Examples of minerals include talc, diamonds, and topaz.

Although a **rock** is also a naturally occurring solid, it can be either organic or inorganic and is composed of one or more minerals. Rocks are classified based on their method of formation. The three types of rocks are igneous, sedimentary, and metamorphic. **Igneous rocks** are the result of tectonic processes that bring magma, or melted rock, to the earth's surface; they can form either above or below the surface. **Sedimentary rocks** are formed from the compaction of rock fragments that results from weathering and erosion. Lastly, **metamorphic rocks** form when extreme temperature and pressure cause the structure of pre-existing rocks to change.

The **rock cycle** describes how rocks form and break down. Typically, the cooling and solidification of magma as it rises to the surface creates igneous rocks. These rocks are then subject to **weathering**, the mechanical and/or chemical processes by which rocks break down. During **erosion** the resulting sediment is deposited in a new location. As sediment is deposited, the resulting compaction creates new sedimentary rocks. As new layers are added, rocks and minerals are forced closer to the earth's core where they are subjected to heat and pressure, resulting in metamorphic rock. Eventually, they will reach their melting point and return to magma, starting the cycle over again. This process takes place over hundreds of thousands or even millions of years.

Paleontology, the study of the history of life on Earth, is sometimes also considered part of geology. Paleontologists study the rock record, which retains biological history through **fossils**, the preserved remains and traces of ancient life. Fossils can be used to learn about the evolution of life on the planet, particularly bacteria, plants, and animals that have gone extinct. Throughout Earth's history, there have been five documented catastrophic events that caused major extinctions. For each mass extinction, there are several theories about the cause but no definitive answers. Theories about what triggered

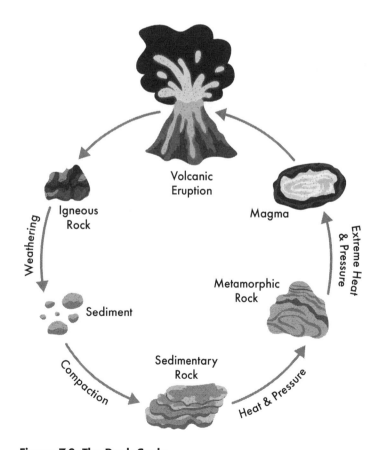

Figure 7.2. The Rock Cycle

mass extinctions include climate change, ice ages, asteroid and comet impacts, and volcanic activity.

The surface of the earth is made of large plates that float on the less dense layer beneath them. These **tectonic plates** make up the lithosphere, the planet's surface layer. Over 200 million years ago, the continents were joined together in one giant landmass called **Pangea**. Due to **continental drift**, or the slow movement of tectonic plates, the continents gradually shifted to their current positions.

> 🔍 Helpful Hint: The magnitude of an earthquake refers to the amount of energy it releases, measured as the maximum motion during the earthquake. This can indirectly describe how destructive the earthquake was.

The boundaries where plates meet are the locations for many geologic features and events. **Mountains** are formed when plates collide and push land upward, and **trenches** form when one plate is pushed beneath another. In addition, the friction created by plates sliding past each other is responsible for most **earthquakes**.

Volcanoes, which are vents in the earth's crust that allow molten rock to reach the surface, frequently occur along the edges of tectonic plates. However, they can also occur at hotspots located far from plate boundaries.

The outermost layer of the earth, which includes tectonic plates, is called the **lithosphere**. Beneath the lithosphere are, in order, the **asthenosphere**, **mesosphere**, and **core**. The core includes two parts: the **outer core** is a liquid layer, and the **inner core** is composed of solid iron. It is believed the inner core spins at a rate slightly different from the rest of the planet, which creates the earth's magnetic field.

PRACTICE QUESTION

2. Rocks are broken down through the process of

   a. fossilization

   b. compaction

   c. sedimentation

   d. erosion

   e. weathering

   Answer:

   e. is correct. Weathering is the process in which rocks are broken down into smaller pieces by physical or chemical means.

Hydrology

The earth's surface includes many bodies of water that together form the **hydrosphere**. The largest of these are the bodies of salt water called **oceans**. There are five oceans: the Arctic,

Atlantic, Indian, Pacific, and Southern. Together, the oceans account for 71 percent of the earth's surface and 97 percent of the earth's water.

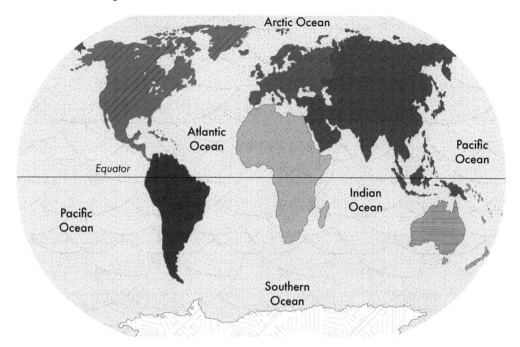

Figure 7.3. The Earth's Oceans

Oceans are subject to cyclic rising and falling water levels at shorelines called **tides**, which are the result of the gravitational pull of the moon and sun. The oceans also experience **waves**, which are caused by the movement of energy through the water.

Other bodies of water include **lakes**, which are usually freshwater, and **seas**, which are usually saltwater. **Rivers** and streams are moving bodies of water that flow into lakes, seas, and oceans. The earth also contains groundwater, or water that is stored underground in rock formations called **aquifers**.

Much of the earth's water is stored as **ice**. The North and South Poles are usually covered in large sheets of ice called polar ice. **Glaciers** are large masses of ice and snow that move. Over long periods of time, they scour Earth's surface, creating features such as lakes and valleys. Large chunks of ice that break off from glaciers are called **icebergs**.

 Did You Know? 97 percent of the water on earth is saltwater. 68 percent of the remaining freshwater is locked up in ice caps and glaciers.

The **water cycle** is the circulation of water throughout the earth's surface, atmosphere, and hydrosphere. Water on the earth's surface evaporates, or changes from a liquid to a gas, and becomes water vapor. Plants also release water vapor through transpiration. Water vapor in the air then comes together to form clouds. When it cools, this water vapor condenses into a liquid and falls from the sky as precipitation, which includes rain, sleet, snow, and hail. Precipitation replenishes groundwater and the water found in features such as lakes and rivers, thus starting the cycle over again.

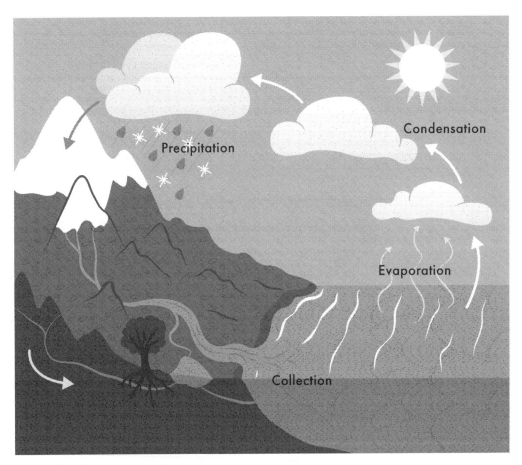

Figure 7.4. The Water Cycle

PRACTICE QUESTION

3. During the water cycle, groundwater is replenished by

    a.   transpiration

    b.   glaciers

    c.   lakes

    d.   precipitation

    e.   evaporation

<u>Answer:</u>

d. is correct. Precipitation such as rain and snow seep into the ground to add to the groundwater supply.

Meteorology

Above the surface of Earth is the mass of gases called the **atmosphere**. The atmosphere includes the **troposphere**, which is closest to the earth, followed by the **stratosphere**, **mesosphere**, and **thermosphere**. The outermost layer of the atmosphere is the **exosphere**, which is located 6,200 miles above the surface. Generally, temperature in the atmosphere decreases with altitude. The **ozone layer**, which captures harmful radiation from the sun, is located in the stratosphere.

> Did You Know? Between each layer, a boundary exists where conditions change. This boundary takes the first part of the name of the previous layer followed by "pause." For example, the boundary between the troposphere and stratosphere is called the tropopause.

The **humidity**, or amount of water vapor in the air, and the **temperature** are two major atmospheric conditions that determine weather, the day-to-day changes in atmospheric conditions. A **warm front** occurs when warm air moves over a cold air mass, causing the air to feel warmer and more humid. A **cold front** occurs when cold air moves under a warm air mass, causing a drop in temperature.

Sometimes, weather turns violent. Tropical cyclones, or hurricanes, originate over warm ocean water. Hurricanes have destructive winds of more than 74 miles per hour and create large storm surges that can cause extensive damage along coastlines. Hurricanes, typhoons, and cyclones are all the same type of storm; they just have different names based on where the storm is located. **Hurricanes** originate in the Atlantic or Eastern Pacific Ocean, **typhoons** in the Western Pacific Ocean, and **cyclones** in the Indian Ocean. **Tornadoes** occur when unstable warm and cold air masses collide and a rotation is created by fast-moving winds.

The long-term weather conditions in a geographic location are called **climate**. A climate zone is a large area that experiences similar average temperature and precipitation. The three major climate zones, based on temperature, are the polar, temperate, and tropical zones. Each climate zone is subdivided into subclimates that have unique characteristics. The **tropical climate zone** (warm temperatures) can be subdivided into tropical wet, tropical wet and dry, semiarid, and arid. The **temperate climate zones** (moderate temperatures) include Mediterranean, humid subtropical, marine West Coast, humid continental, and subarctic. The **polar climate zones** (cold temperatures) include tundra, highlands, nonpermanent ice, and ice cap. Polar climates are cold and experience prolonged, dark winters due to the tilt of the earth's axis.

PRACTICE QUESTION

4. The layer of the atmosphere that absorbs harmful ultraviolet radiation from the sun is the

   a. mesosphere

   b. stratosphere

   c. troposphere

   d. thermosphere

   e. exosphere

<u>Answer:</u>

b. is correct. The stratosphere contains a sublayer called the ozone layer, which absorbs harmful ultraviolet radiation from the sun.

Test Your Knowledge

Read the question, and then choose the most correct answer.

1. Which planet orbits closest to Earth?

   a. Mercury

   b. Venus

   c. Jupiter

   d. Saturn

2. What is the name of the phenomenon when a star suddenly increases in brightness and then disappears from view?

   a. aurora

   b. black hole

   c. eclipse

   d. supernova

3. How long does it take the earth to rotate on its axis?

   a. one hour

   b. one day

   c. one month

   d. one year

4. Which statement about the solar system is true?

   a. Earth is much closer to the sun than it is to other stars.

   b. The moon is closer to Venus than it is to Earth.

   c. At certain times of the year, Jupiter is closer to the sun than Earth is.

   d. Mercury is the closest planet to Earth.

5. When Earth moves between the moon and the sun, it is called a

   a. solar eclipse.

   b. lunar eclipse.

   c. black hole.

   d. supernova.

6. Which planet does not have a moon?

   a. Mercury

   b. Earth

   c. Jupiter

   d. Saturn

7. What is the term for the top layer of the earth's surface?

   a. lithosphere

   b. atmosphere

   c. biosphere

   d. asthenosphere

8. Which action is an example of mechanical weathering?

   a. Calcium carbonate reacts with water to form a cave.

   b. An iron gate rusts.

   c. Tree roots grow under the foundation of a house and cause cracks.

   d. Feldspar turns to clay when exposed to water.

9. Which of the following is caused by geothermal heat?

   a. geysers

   b. tsunamis

   c. tornadoes

   d. hurricanes

10. Which of the following holds the largest percentage of the earth's freshwater?

   a. glaciers and ice caps
   b. groundwater
   c. lakes
   d. oceans

11. Which of the following best describes how igneous rocks are formed?

   a. Sediment is compacted by pressure in the earth to form rock.
   b. Magma comes to the earth's surface and cools to form rock.
   c. Chemical weathering changes the composition of a rock to form new rock.
   d. Ancient plant and animal life is calcified to create rock.

12. Which of the following is true as altitude increases in the troposphere?

   a. Temperature and pressure increase.
   b. Temperature increases and pressure decreases.
   c. Temperature and pressure decrease.
   d. Temperature decreases and pressure increases.

13. Which statement about hurricanes and tornadoes is true?

   a. Hurricanes and tornadoes spin in opposite directions.
   b. Tornadoes do not occur in warm climates.
   c. Tornadoes have a low wind velocity.
   d. Hurricanes are formed over warm ocean water.

14. Which two properties are used to classify climate zones?

   a. latitude and temperature
   b. temperature and precipitation
   c. elevation and latitude
   d. precipitation and tilt of Earth's axis

15. Which of the following best describes continental drift?

   a. The mass extinction of the earth's species that occurred when a meteor struck the earth.
   b. The spinning of the earth's inner core that creates the earth's magnetic field.
   c. The formation of land masses from cooled magma.
   d. The movement of tectonic plates in the lithosphere.

ANSWER KEY

1. **b.**

   Venus's orbit is closest to Earth and is the second planet from the sun.

2. **d.**

   Before a star collapses, the star burns brighter for a period of time and then fades from view. This is a supernova.

3. **b.**

   Earth takes approximately twenty-four hours to rotate on its axis.

4. **a.**

   The sun is about ninety-three million miles from Earth; the next closest star is about twenty-five trillion miles away.

5. **b.**

   A lunar eclipse is when Earth moves between the moon and the sun.

6. **a.**

   Only the first two planets, Mercury and Venus, lack moons.

7. **a.**

   The lithosphere is the top layer of the earth's surface.

8. **c.**

   Mechanical weathering involves breaking a substance down without changing the composition of the substance.

9. **a.**

   Geysers are caused by geothermal heating of water underground.

10. **a.**

    Glaciers and ice caps contain approximately 68.7% of all of Earth's freshwater supply, which is the largest percentage of the resources listed.

11. **b.**

    Igneous rock is formed when magma (melted rock) is brought to the earth's surface and cools.

12. **c.**

    Temperature and pressure both decrease with altitude in the troposphere.

13. **d.**

    Hurricanes require warm ocean water to form.

14. **b.**

    Climate zones are classified by temperature and precipitation.

15. **d.**

    Continental drift is the movement of tectonic plates that lead to the current position of the continents.

EIGHT: JUDGMENT AND COMPREHENSION

The questions on the Judgment and Comprehension in Practical Nursing Situations test will assess your understanding of the role of the practice nurse in the workplace. Each question will present a workplace scenario and four possible responses. You will need to pick the response that is most appropriate for a practical nurse in a professional setting.

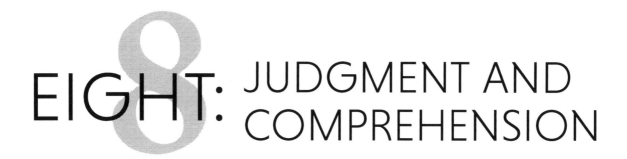

Judgment and Comprehension in Practical Nursing Situations Question Format

In this part, there are a number of questions about the working relationships of the practical and vocational nurse. Each work situation is followed by four possible answers to the problem presented. Select the one answer that, in your judgment, is the best of the four.

While you are performing an intake exam, the patient asks if you think he has a kidney stone. How should the practical nurse respond?

a.   "Let me help you figure out what's wrong."

b.   "I am not experienced enough to know."

c.   "You are not supposed to ask me that."

d.   "Only a doctor can offer a diagnosis."

Scope of Practice for the Practical Nurse

The practical nurse (PN) is found in a number of health care settings as an assistant or adjunct to the registered nurse (RN) or physician/provider. A practical nurse may work in any health care setting, including hospitals, long-term care, home care, or clinics. They will be responsible for the delegated tasks assigned to them that are within their scope of practice. Important qualities of practical nurses include reliability, adaptability, organizational skills, and communication skills.

Scope of practice for PNs is governed by the state board of nursing and may also be limited by the PN's employer. The scope of practice varies from state to state, but in general PNs will be responsible for stable patients who require routine care. Possible tasks may include:

+ taking routine vital signs

+ helping patients with activities of daily living (ADL)

+ administering medications

+ collecting specimens

+ caring for wounds, catheters, and feeding tubes

+ setting up basic equipment

PNs should not perform any tasks that require diagnosing or planning care and should not be responsible for unstable patients. Tasks that are always **outside** the PN's scope of practice include:

+ diagnosing medical conditions

+ developing or changing plans of care

+ educating patients (except for routine tasks such as handwashing)

+ administering push IV medication or blood products

It is the practical nurse's responsibility to know their own scope of practice. The nurse should notify the registered nurse or physician if the duties they have been assigned violate their scope of practice: DO NOT assume that those delegating tasks know the PN's scope of practice. Such communication should be respectful and professional to preserve the working relationship of the health care team. Physician consent is required before the practical nurse can perform any intervention that is invasive or includes tasks not normally initiated by the practical nurse (e.g., Foley catheter placement).

Therapeutic Communication

Therapeutic communication is a set of techniques used to communicate with patients that addresses the physical, mental, and emotional well-being of patients. The goal of therapeutic communication is to build a strong nurse-patient relationship. Important aspects of therapeutic communication include:

+ **Show acceptance of the patient.** Do not judge patients or argue with their choices.

+ **Address patient concerns with respect and consideration.** When patients express concern regarding their care, the practical nurse should acknowledge that concern and actively listen to the patient.

+ **Remain calm in the face of aggressive behavior.** In health care settings, patients or their families may be aggressive, violent, or disrespectful to the nurse. When these situations occur, the PN should inform the patient that type of behavior is not acceptable. If the PN feels unsafe or cannot complete their work, they should report the behavior to the RN or physician in charge.

+ **Avoid negative communication techniques.** Do not use medical jargon that could confuse the patient, give unwanted advice, or act defensive when questioned by a patient.

Reporting to the Supervisor

The PN always works under direct supervision, usually under an RN, a physician, or a physician's assistant (PA). The PN should keep an open line of communication with their supervisor and report to them as needed. Situations that should always be reported to supervisors include:

+ patient concerns and questions
+ changes in patient condition
+ errors made by the PN
+ errors witnessed by the PN
+ staff misbehavior

Privacy

The PN should make sure that communication in a health care setting protects the privacy of patients, their families, and staff members. Some guidelines for privacy are given below.

+ Do not discuss patients' private health information in public spaces.
+ Do not discuss sensitive information about coworkers in public spaces.
+ Only share information with other health care providers that is necessary for medical care.
+ Do not discuss patients with other patients or their families.
+ Only share information about patients with people approved by that patient.

Test Your Knowledge

Read the question, and then choose the most correct answer.

1. A patient makes discriminatory comments about the race of the nurse's assistant behind his back. The most appropriate response is to:

    a.   say, "Sir, your comments are disgusting. I am going to refuse my services if you continue."

    b.   say, "Sir, you need to be quiet, or I am going to tell him exactly what you said."

    c.   say nothing and report the incident to the police for proper documentation.

    d.   say nothing and ignore the behavior; document the incident if it escalates to threats or interpersonal aggression.

2. You see a coworker drinking on the job. You should:

    a.   report the incident immediately to a supervisor.

    b.   mind your own business.

    c.   respectfully confront the coworker.

    d.   brainstorm the best approach with another coworker.

3. You are working in a physician's office that allows only one family member to accompany a patient for a checkup. A family of five is trying to crowd into the checkup room. You politely explain the rules and ask them to leave, but they refuse. The best thing to do is:

    a.   call the police.

    b.   tell the family off.

    c.   contact a supervisor for instructions.

    d.   ask another patient's family to assist.

4. An elderly patient with severe health issues is refusing to take his medications. What should the practical nurse do?

    a.   Do not ask questions—it is the patient's right to refuse.

    b.   Help the patient by throwing away the medications.

    c.   Ask the patient why he is refusing the medications.

    d.   Call a supervisor immediately because it is an emergency.

5. A patient is due for a daily bath and tells you he's never had anyone help him bathe before. You should:

    a.   start the bath immediately and tell the patient to undress.

    b.   explain that the bath is mandatory, and you have been told to assist.

    c.   tell the patient not to worry because nurses see nude people all the time.

    d.   explain each step and why you are doing it.

ANSWER KEY

1.   **d.**

   The best approach is to document the behavior and then notify a supervisor. A police report would not be appropriate, and threatening the patient will likely escalate the behavior.

2.   **a.**

   All nurses and medical providers are ethically obligated to report such behavior to the board of nursing or other credentialing bodies immediately. Confronting the coworker or brainstorming with others are not appropriate actions. Ignoring the issue is unethical.

3.   **c.**

   This situation may require a supervisor to back you up and compel the family members to leave the room. The police have no jurisdiction or role in this situation, nor does another patient's family.

4.   **c.**

   The practical nurse should discuss this issue with the patient and help him understand why compliance is important. A supervisor should not be necessary in this case. It is not appropriate to ignore the issue or discard the medications.

5.   **d.**

   Due to the sensitive nature of bathing a patient, it is important to be in constant communication. Treating a patient with dignity and respect is paramount. The remaining options are not conducive to patient dignity and respect.

NINE: VOCATIONAL ADJUSTMENT INDEX

The ninety questions on the Vocational Adjustment Index assess your personal attitudes, characteristics, and behaviors. Schools will use your score on this section to assess whether your personality is a fit for health care occupations.

Each question is a simple, general statement about personal or professional situations. You will choose to agree or disagree with the statement. You will need to work quickly to answer all the questions.

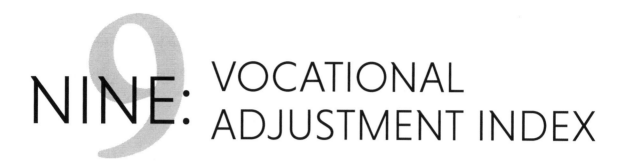

Vocational Adjustment Index Question Format

The following statements address certain personal or professional situations. Agreeing or disagreeing with the statements simply reveals how you are likely to think, feel, or act in certain circumstances. If you agree with the statement, select (A) in the corresponding row. If you disagree, select (D). Choose the answer that is most true for you and answer immediately. Work rapidly.

1.	It is more important to be accurate than to be on time.	(A)	(D)
2.	An ideal job includes a flexible schedule.	(A)	(D)
3.	People who act like my friends have betrayed me.	(A)	(D)
4.	It is difficult to make decisions in stressful situations.	(A)	(D)
5.	Many people spend too much time on their phones.	(A)	(D)

There are no right or wrong answers, so there is no need to waste time deciding what the answer *should* be. Some statements are unflattering or critical, so it might be uncomfortable to select one. That is okay; it is best to answer as honestly as possible. You should also keep in mind that the chosen answers are not meant to be statements of fact. You don't have to select an answer that is necessarily a true statement about yourself, just the one that most generally applies to you.

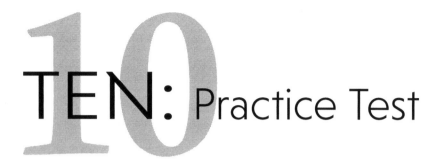

TEN: Practice Test

ACADEMIC APTITUDE: VERBAL SKILLS

Which word is most different in meaning from the other words?

1.	a. distressed	b. worried	c. calm	d. anxious	e. stressed
2.	a. tired	b. exhausted	c. lazy	d. weary	e. energetic
3.	a. problem	b. complication	c. difficulty	d. certainty	e. obstacle
4.	a. mythical	b. ordinary	c. miraculous	d. magical	e. different
5.	a. rot	b. wither	c. thrive	d. fail	e. struggle
6.	a. attentive	b. thoughtless	c. responsible	d. caring	e. considerate
7.	a. complete	b. thorough	c. lacking	d. exhaustive	e. full
8.	a. laceration	b. scrape	c. bandage	d. wound	e. sore
9.	a. lively	b. dull	c. gloomy	d. somber	e. unhappy
10.	a. brief	b. terse	c. concise	d. long	e. sudden
11.	a. secretive	b. obscure	c. mysterious	d. cryptic	e. obvious
12.	a. gloomy	b. upbeat	c. irritable	d. glum	e. moody
13.	a. obsession	b. attraction	c. passion	d. interest	e. indifference
14.	a. pleasant	b. amiable	c. kindly	d. cheerful	e. rude
15.	a. combine	b. connect	c. join	d. divide	e. unite
16.	a. destroy	b. finish	c. create	d. shatter	e. ruin
17.	a. cascade	b. drip	c. torrent	d. flood	e. surge

18.   a. calm   b. quiet   c. conflict   d. peace   e. order

19.   a. limited   b. endless   c. eternal   d. lasting   e. constant

20.   a. acquit   b. excuse   c. pardon   d. disapprove   e. absolve

21.   a. arrogance   b. humility   c. vanity   d. narcissism   e. smugness

22.   a. weak   b. defective   c. broken   d. flawed   e. perfect

23.   a. humble   b. bashful   c. timid   d. conceited   e. modest

24.   a. civil   b. polite   c. refined   d. crude   e. gracious

25.   a. absurd   b. playful   c. foolish   d. silly   e. serious

ACADEMIC APTITUDE: ARITHMETIC

Work the problem, and then choose the correct answer.

---

26. Danika bought two packages of ground beef weighing 1.73 lb and 2.17 lb. What was the total weight of the two packages in pounds?

a. 0.44   b. 1.25   c. 3.81   d. 3.9   e. 4.2

27. Morris went shopping with $80. He spent $24.17 at the hardware store and $32.87 on clothes. How much money did he have left?

a. $22.96   b. $23.04   c. $42.96   d. $55.83   e. $57.04

28. What is the remainder when 397 is divided by 4?

a. 0   b. 1   c. 2   d. 3   e. 4

29. A teacher has 50 notebooks to hand out to students. If she has 16 students in her class, and each student receives 2 notebooks, how many notebooks will she have left over?

a. 2   b. 16   c. 18   d. 32   e. 34

30. Michael is making cupcakes. He plans to give $\frac{1}{2}$ of the cupcakes to a friend and $\frac{1}{3}$ of the cupcakes to his coworkers. If he makes 48 cupcakes, how many will he have left over?

a. 8   b. 10   c. 12   d. 16   e. 24

31. Which of the following is closest in value to 129,113 + 34,602?

a. 162,000   b. 163,000   c. 164,000   d. 165,000   e. 166,000

32. Students board a bus at 7:45 a.m. and arrive at school at 8:20 a.m. For how many minutes are the students on the bus?

a. 30   b. 35   c. 45   d. 50   e. 65

33. Micah has invited 23 friends to his house and is having pizza for dinner. If each pizza feeds 4 people, how many pizzas should he order?

a. 4   b. 5   c. 6   d. 7   e. 8

34. Out of 1,560 students at Ward Middle School, 15% want to take French. Which expression represents how many students want to take French?

a. 1560 ÷ 15   b. 1560 × 15   c. 1560 × 1.51   d. 1560 ÷ 0.15   e. 1560 × 0.15

35. At the grocery store, apples cost $1.89 per pound and oranges cost $2.19 per pound. How much would it cost to purchase 2 lb of apples and 1.5 lb of oranges?

a. $6.62   b. $7.07   c. $7.14   d. $7.22   e. $7.67

36. Which digit is in the hundredths place when 1.3208 is divided by 5.2?

    a. 0   b. 4   c. 5   d. 8   e. 9

37. 17.38 − 19.26 + 14.2 =

    a. 12.08   b. 12.32   c. 16.08   d. 16.22   e. 50.84

38. If a person reads 40 pages in 45 minutes, approximately how many minutes will it take her to read 265 pages?

    a. 180   b. 202   c. 236   d. 265   e. 298

39. The recommended ratio of nurses to patients in a critical care unit is 1 to 4. How many nurses should be on duty if there are 20 patients in the unit?

    a. 4   b. 5   c. 7   d. 8   e. 10

40. Jim is taking care of eight patients during his shift. So far it has taken him 25 minutes to see two patients. At this rate, how many minutes will it take Jim to check in on all eight patients?

    a. 50   b. 60   c. 100   d. 120   e. 125

41. Juan is packing a shipment of three books weighing 0.8 lb, 0.49 lb, and 0.89 lb. The maximum weight for the shipping box is 2.5 lb. How much more weight will the box hold in pounds?

    a. 0.32   b. 0.48   c. 1.61   d. 2.18   e. 4.68

42. The average rainfall in May for Austin, Texas, is 4.5 in. In July, the average rainfall is 1.67 in. How many more inches of rain fall on average in May than in July?

    a. 1.22   b. 2.69   c. 2.83   d. 2.97   e. 6.17

43. If a $285.48 bill will be split evenly between six people, how much will each person pay?

    a. $47.58   b. $49.88   c. $225.48   d. $885.46   e. $1,712.88

44. A bridge is 119.7 m long in the summer. In the winter, the metal contracts, and the bridge shrinks by 1.05 m. How many meters long is the bridge in winter?

    a. 109.2   b. 118.2   c. 118.65   d. 120.75   e. 130.2

45. Angelica bought a roast weighing 3.2 lb. If the roast cost $25.44, how much did it cost per pound?

    a. $5.95   b. $7.44   c. $7.95   d. $8.14   e. $22.24

46. A box of books weighs 6.3 lb. If there are 18 books in the box, how many pounds does each book weigh?

    a. 0.35   b. 1.134   c. 3.5   d. 11.34   e. 35

47. Carlos spent $1.68 on bananas. If bananas cost 48 cents per pound, how many pounds of bananas did he buy?

    a. 1.2   b. 2.06   c. 2.16   d. 3.5   e. 8.1

48. Sally has $127 in her checking. An automatic draft takes out $150 for her electric bill. What is her balance after the automatic draft?

    a. −$277   b. −$123   c. −$23   d. $23   e. $123

49. Five numbers have an average of 16. If the first four numbers have a sum of 68, what is the fifth number?

    a. 12   b. 16   c. 52   d. 68   e. 80

50. The recommended dosage of a particular medication is 4 mL per 50 lb of body weight. What is the recommended dosage in milliliters for a person who weighs 175 lb?

    a. 14   b. 25   c. 28   d. 44   e. 140

ACADEMIC APTITUDE: NONVERBAL SKILLS

Which shape correctly completes the statement?

51. △ is to ⚠ as ◇ is to ?

a. ▽ b. ◈ c. ◈ d. ▢ e. ◈

52. ⋈ is to ◁ as ◖ is to ?

a. △ b. ◇ c. ◗ d. ◁ e. ○

53. ⬡ is to ⬢ as △ is to ?

a. ● b. ▲ c. ■ d. ◆ e. ◀

54. ◔ is to ◔ as ◔ is to ?

a. ◔ b. ◕ c. ◔ d. ◕ e. ◔

55. 8 is to 8 as 8 is to ?

a. 8 b. 8 c. 8 d. 8 e. 8

56. ◩ is to ⋈ as ◪ is to ?

a. ◺ b. ◀ c. ⋈ d. ◩ e. ◪

57. ⠙ is to ⠄ as ⠆ is to ?

a. ⠤ b. ⠛ c. ⠶ d. ⠌ e. ⠄

58. ⊟ is to ⊟ as ⊟ is to ?

a. ⊟ b. ⊟ c. ⊐ d. ⊟ e. ⊟

59. ‖‖‖ is to |‖‖ as ‖‖‖ is to ?

a. ⫴ b. ⫴ c. ⫴ d. ⫴ e. ⫴

60. ⊔ is to ⊔ as ⊏ is to ?

a. ⊩ b. ⊏ c. ⊏ d. ⊩ e. ⊏

61. ◕ is to ◔ as ◔ is to ?

a. ◔ b. ◔ c. ◔ d. ◔ e. ◔

62. ⌐ is to ⌐ as ⌐ is to ?

a. ⊓ b. ⊓ c. ⊓ d. ⊓ e. ⊓

63. ⊞ is to ⊞ as ◩ is to ?

a. ◸ b. ⊞ c. ◹ d. ⊞ e. ⊠

64. ╱ is to ⌒ as ⌐ is to ?

a. ⌂ b. ⌐ c. ⊓ d. ⊔ e. ⬠

65. ⬓ is to ⬓ as ⬓ is to ?

a. ⬓ b. ⬓ c. ⬓ d. ⬓ e. ⬓

66. ▢ is to ▢ as ▢ is to ?

a. ▢ b. ▢ c. ▢ d. ▢ e. ▢

67. ◆◆ is to ◆◆ as ◆◆ is to ?

a. ◆◆ b. ◆◆ c. ◆ d. ◆◆ e. ◆◆

68. (x) is to (x) as (x) is to ?

a. (+) b. (x) c. (+) d. (x) e. (x)

69. ‖‖ is to ‖‖ as ‖‖ is to ?

a. ‖‖ b. ‖‖ c. ‖‖ d. ‖‖ e. ‖‖

70. ✕ is to ✕ as ✕ is to ?

a. ✕ b. ✕ c. ✕ d. ✕ e. ✕

71. ▫ is to ⊏ as ⌐ is to ?

a. ⅂ b. ⅃ c. ═ d. ⎸ e. ⊔

72. (x) is to (x) as (x) is to ?

a. (x) b. (x) c. (x) d. (+) e. (x)

73. ▫ is to ▪ as ◿ is to ?

a. ◢ b. ◣ c. ◢ d. ▲ e. ◺

74. ⬚ is to ⬚ as ⬚ is to ?

a. ⬚ b. ⬚ c. ⬚ d. ⬚ e. ⬚

75. ⅃ is to L as ⌐ is to ?

a. L b. ⌐ c. ⌐ d. ⅃ e. ⌐

SPELLING

Choose the correct spelling of the word.

1. a. muscle   b. muscle   c. mucsel
2. a. hormoan   b. hormmone   c. hormone
3. a. seesure   b. seizure   c. seazure
4. a. facilitees   b. facilitys   c. facilities
5. a. decrease   b. decreese   c. decreace
6. a. transfusion   b. transfussion   c. transfution
7. a. annatome   b. anatomy   c. annatomy
8. a. daignoses   b. diagnosis   c. diegnosis
9. a. equepment   b. equipmint   c. equipment
10. a. stomach   b. stomache   c. stomeche
11. a. athritis   b. arthritis   c. arthritise
12. a. overy   b. ovary   c. ovarry
13. a. surgical   b. surgicle   c. sergical
14. a. allerjy   b. alerrgy   c. allergy
15. a. inflammation   b. enflamation   c. inflamation
16. a. poisson   b. pioson   c. poison
17. a. atrophy   b. attrophy   c. atrophe
18. a. stierile   b. sterile   c. steerile
19. a. cellular   b. celullar   c. celluler
20. a. tisue   b. tissue   c. tissu
21. a. artifitial   b. artificial   c. artifacial
22. a. immediet   b. immidiate   c. immediate
23. a. droplat   b. dropplet   c. droplet
24. a. symptom   b. symptome   c. simptom
25. a. eleminate   b. elemenate   c. eliminate
26. a. adhear   b. adhere   c. adher

27. a. inable   b. enable   c. ennable

28. a. varyous   b. various   c. variouse

29. a. secression   b. secresion   c. secretion

30. a. traumma   b. traumme   c. trauma

31. a. exsessive   b. excesive   c. excessive

32. a. bacteria   b. bactieria   c. bactteria

33. a. funngas   b. funngus   c. fungus

34. a. monetor   b. monitor   c. moniter

35. a. abration   b. abrassion   c. abrasion

36. a. multipal   b. multipple   c. multiple

37. a. tremor   b. tremer   c. tremour

38. a. involvment   b. envolvement   c. involvement

39. a. respiritory b. resperitory   c. respiratory

40. a. craneal   b. cranial   c. crannial

41. a. dissease   b. diseasse   c. disease

42. a. artery   b. arttery   c. arterie

43. a. vaine   b. vein   c. veine

44. a. cronic   b. chronic   c. chronick

45. a. accute   b. acutte   c. acute

GENERAL SCIENCE

Read the question, and then choose the most correct answer.

1. The inorganic material that makes up bone is

    a. calcium   b. phosphorus   c. collagen   d. potassium   e. actin

2. An example of a biome is a

    a. beehive   b. cornfield   c. herd of bison   d. desert   e. puddle

3. The planet that is closest to Earth is

    a. Mercury   b. Venus   c. Jupiter   d. Saturn   e. Neptune

4. The phenomenon when a star suddenly increases in brightness and then disappears from view is a(n)

    a. aurora   b. galaxy   c. black hole   d. eclipse   e. supernova

5. Chloroplasts can be found in the cells of

    a. whales   b. mushrooms   c. tulips   d. lizards   e. fish

6. Isotopes of an element will have the same number of

    a. electrons   b. neutrons   c. protons   d. atoms   e. ions

7. An electrocardiogram (EKG) can be used to diagnose

    a. diabetes   b. torn ligaments   c. cancer   d. tachycardia   e. influenza

8. The number of nucleotides in a codon is

    a. 3   b. 4   c. 6   d. 22   e. 64

9. The negatively charged atoms inside an atom are called

    a. protons   b. neutrons   c. electrons   d. ions   e. nucleus

10. A box sliding down a ramp experiences all of the following forces EXCEPT

    a. tension   b. friction   c. gravity   d. normal   e. buoyant

11. An example of an organism that decomposes organic matter is a(n)

   a. apple tree   b. mushroom   c. goat   d. lion   e. vulture

12. An example of an organism that regulates its body temperature externally is a

   a. pelican   b. dolphin   c. whale   d. lobster   e. leopard

13. Which part of the body is affected by a right tibia fracture?

   a. upper arm   b. lower arm   c. upper leg   d. lower leg   e. head

14. The digestive enzymes produced by the pancreas pass into the

   a. stomach   b. gallbladder   c. esophagus   d. large intestine   e. small intestine

15. An example of a physical change is

   a. freezing water   b. baking a cake   c. a rusting fence   d. an exploding firecracker   e. neutralizing an acid

16. A nonrenewable energy source is

   a. water   b. wind   c. coal   d. sunlight   e. geothermal

17. The top layer of the earth's surface is called the

   a. exosphere   b. lithosphere   c. atmosphere   d. biosphere   e. asthenosphere

18. Skeletal muscle is attached to bone by

   a. ligaments   b. cartilage   c. tendons   d. nerves   e. fascia

19. During digestion, food passes through the

   a. esophagus   b. gallbladder   c. trachea   d. pancreas   e. liver

20. The earth rotates on its axis in

   a. one hour   b. one day   c. one month   d. one year   e. one hundred years

21. The process that uses carbon dioxide to produce sugars is called

   a. digestion   b. chloroplast   c. decomposition   d. photosynthesis   e. cellular respiration

22. $2C_6H_{14} + 19O_2 \rightarrow 12CO_2 + 14H_2O$

The reaction shown above is a(n)

a. substitution reaction
b. acid-base reaction
c. decomposition reaction
d. combustion reaction
e. synthesis reaction

23. The abiotic factor in an ecosystem could include

a. producers
b. consumers
c. predators
d. decomposers
e. water

24. In a food web, fungi are

a. producers
b. primary consumers
c. secondary consumers
d. tertiary consumers
e. decomposers

25. The mechanism of evolution is

a. gene flow
b. genetic drift
c. mutation
d. sexual selection
e. natural selection

26. The muscular organ that processes food material into smaller pieces and helps mix it with saliva is the

a. pharynx
b. tongue
c. diaphragm
d. stomach
e. esophagus

27. A strong acid will

a. completely ionize in water
b. donate more than one proton
c. have a pH close to 7
d. not ionize
e. have at least one metal atom

28. The largest bone in the human body is the

a. tibia
b. humerus
c. scapula
d. femur
e. ulna

29. When skin is exposed to the sunlight, it produces

a. vitamin A
b. vitamin E
c. vitamin K
d. vitamin D
e. vitamin B

30. The light reactions of photosynthesis occur in the

a. mitochondria
b. chloroplast
c. cytoplasm
d. vacuole
e. nucleus

31. The exchange of nutrients, gases, and cellular waste happens in the

a. veins
b. arteries
c. capillaries
d. venules
e. arterioles

32. The incus, stapes, and malleus play an important role in

   a. vision   b. taste   c. hearing   d. smell   e. touch

33. The adrenal glands are located near the

   a. brain   b. thyroid   c. kidneys   d. bladder   e. heart

34. Wind speed is measured using

   a. a thermometer   b. a wind vane   c. an anemometer   d. a rain gauge   e. a barometer

35. One milliliter is equivalent to

   a. 1 g   b. 1 pt   c. 1 lb   d. 1 m^2 e. 1 cm^3

36. Mature sperm is stored in the

   a. testes   b. bladder   c. vas deferens   d. epididymis   e. penis

37. The meninges protect the

   a. brain   b. heart   c. stomach   d. uterus   e. testes

38. Organic molecules must contain

   a. carbon   b. phosphorous   c. nitrogen   d. oxygen   e. helium

39. DNA and RNA are built from monomers called

   a. amino acids   b. sugars   c. lipids   d. polymerases   e. nucleotides

40. The nucleotide found in RNA but not DNA is

   a. adenine   b. cytosine   c. thymine   d. uracil   e. guanine

41. An organism with 16 total chromosomes will produce gametes with a chromosome number of

   a. 4   b. 8   c. 16   d. 32   e. 64

42. An example of a wedge is a(n)

   a. wagon   b. ramp   c. ax   d. seesaw   e. car axle

43. The number of electrons needed by a noble gas to fill its outermost electron shell is

   a. 0   b. 1   c. 2   d. 3   e. 4

44. Photosynthesis takes place in the

   a. roots   b. stem   c. bark   d. flower   e. leaves

45. The process that occurs when water vapor becomes a solid is

   a. condensation   b. sublimation   c. evaporation   d. deposition   e. freezing

46. Orange juice, which is primarily composed of citric acid and malic acid, likely has a pH of

   a. 4   b. 7   c. 9   d. 13   e. 14

47. The mass of an object is measured with a

   a. thermometer   b. graduated cylinder   c. ruler   d. barometer   e. balance

48. The resistance to motion caused by one object rubbing against another object is

   a. inertia   b. friction   c. velocity   d. gravity   e. acceleration

49. The rock formed when lava cools and solidifies is called

   a. igneous   b. sedimentary   c. metamorphic   d. sandstone   e. mineral

50. An example of a longitudinal wave is a

   a. surface wave   b. light wave   c. sound wave   d. radio wave   e. microwave

51. The gas found in the largest quantity in Earth's atmosphere is

   a. carbon monoxide   b. bromine   c. nitrogen   d. fluorine   e. oxygen

52. All atoms of an element contain the same number of

   a. electrons   b. molecules   c. protons   d. ions   e. neutrons

53. The most common element in the universe is

   a. carbon   b. lithium   c. potassium   d. titanium   e. hydrogen

54. The storm LEAST likely to form over ocean water is a

    a. hurricane   b. typhoon   c. cyclone   d. tornado   e. squall

55. To neutralize an acid spill, use

    a. baking soda   b. lemon juice   c. cat litter   d. water   e. vinegar

56. The force that attracts a body toward the center of the earth is

    a. friction   b. gravity   c. pull   d. tension   e. buoyancy

57. Energy that is stored and is waiting to work is called

    a. kinetic   b. thermal   c. mechanical   d. chemical   e. potential

58. An example of a translucent object is a

    a. book   b. glass of water   c. T-shirt   d. car window   e. door

59. An example of an electrical insulator is a

    a. spoon   b. key   c. marble   d. penny   e. wire

60. Stratus clouds can be described as

    a. often gray   b. big and tall   c. high in the sky   d. puffy   e. usually wispy

JUDGMENT AND COMPREHENSION

Read the question, and then choose the most correct answer.

---

1. Lately your paperwork has not been in compliance because you feel too stressed on the job. What should you do?

    a. Outsource the paperwork to an assistant

    b. Set up an appointment with your supervisor

    c. Ask your coworker to help you

    d. Just keep trying your best

2. Another nurse keeps shifting her duties your way, which is making you feel overwhelmed. You should:

    a. Call HR

    b. Tell her she needs to stop being lazy

    c. Have a private meeting to explain that you can no longer assist her

    d. Keep helping her so her work gets done correctly

3. Another employee asks you to cover for him while he makes a quick run to the store. You should:

    a. Politely deny the request

    b. Tell him to find someone who is as incompetent as he is

    c. Threaten him with an HR report

    d. Ask your nurse's assistant to cover for him

4. A child keeps throwing water next to a patient's medical machine. The parent is not intervening. You should tell the parent:

    a. "You need to teach your child some manners."

    b. "Are you just going to sit there and do nothing?"

    c. "Do you need some parental counseling? Your child is clearly breaching safety protocols here."

    d. "Throwing water around the medical equipment can be dangerous. Can you please ask your child to stop?"

5. A patient with a broken arm tells you he is scared. You should respond by saying:

    a. "There is no need to worry. Your arm will be fine."

    b. "It is not that bad. I would stop worrying."

    c. "I understand. Is there anything I can do to help?"

    d. "You are embarrassing yourself."

6. A grieving mother demands to see the patient who crashed into her son's car. You should:

    a. Deny the request and withhold any information

    b. Let her handle the situation

    c. Call the police on her

    d. Ask the patient if they would like to see the woman

7. You are not feeling well and are unsure about the procedures for taking a sick day. You should:

   a. Just take off without notification because you are ill
   b. Review any training materials and contact your supervisor if necessary
   c. Go in to work to ask what to do
   d. Text a coworker to tell your supervisor

8. A patient tells you that the pain medication you gave him is making him feel anxious. Your response should be:

   a. "I am here to help. Let me check with the practitioner."
   b. "I think you are having an allergic reaction. I can help."
   c. "A lot of medications have adverse effects on patients."
   d. "You are probably just a little delirious from pain medications."

9. You were trained on a certain procedure but have forgotten how to carry it out properly. You should:

   a. Try your best to remember
   b. Ask a fellow nurse to show you
   c. Ask your supervisor for assistance
   d. Tell your supervisor not to assign you to the procedure

10. A fellow nurse is just sitting around instead of doing work. You should:

    a. Take a photo for evidence
    b. Call security
    c. Discuss the issue with the lead nurse
    d. Tell her she is lazy

11. An angry patient demands the personal email of your supervisor. You should:

    a. Tell him that is a ridiculous request
    b. Give him a fake email
    c. Connect him with patient relations
    d. Give him your email instead

12. Due to your negligence, a young patient slips in the bathroom. You and the patient are alone, without any witnesses. You should:

    a. Call a lawyer immediately
    b. Call the supervising nurse
    c. Leave the scene
    d. Ask a visitor for assistance

13. A patient is feeling self-conscious about the IV they have to walk around with. You can help the situation by saying:

    a. "Nobody cares."
    b. "It is normal to feel this way, but the IV is helping you."
    c. "Just forget about it."
    d. "You are overreacting."

14. How should you treat a child with a terminal brain tumor?

a. You should make exceptions to rules

b. You should help normalize the environment by treating them like any other patient

c. You should talk to them directly about the tumor

d. You should counsel them through prayer

15. A patient in the clinic is complaining of stomach pain. You should:

a. Help diagnose the problem

b. Ask the patient about the nature and characteristics of the pain

c. Put on the TV to distract the patient from the pain

d. Tell the patient about what possible illnesses they could be experiencing

16. A patient's aunt, who is also a nurse, says she wants to give him some pain pills. You should tell her:

a. She needs to provide her credentials

b. That is a stupid suggestion, and she should know that because she is a nurse

c. She needs to refrain from making suggestions because it goes against protocols

d. That is not acceptable, and she will need to leave the room

17. In order to achieve all goals in the workplace as a nurse, you must:

a. Experiment with new ideas

b. Be flexible when it comes to procedures

c. Put customer service first

d. Have a thorough understanding of the nursing profession

18. Your supervisor says it is going to be a busy day at work. He assigns you a list of duties that is twice as long as your regular list. You do not think you will be able to complete all the duties. You should:

a. Try, knowing you will fail

b. Request a private meeting to discuss the matter

c. Tell your supervisor he is expecting too much

d. Find a job that is not as demanding

19. One of your duties as a nurse is helping a patient go to the bathroom. You should:

a. Give a step-by-step explanation of what you are doing and why

b. Lighten up the uncomfortable situation by making the patient laugh

c. Tell the patient that this is a normal, everyday task

d. Go through the process without saying anything in order to avoid any awkwardness

20. In a moment of crisis, a supervisor asks you to break an important institutional protocol. You should:

  a. Quit on the spot   b. Contact a legal representative   c. Remind her of the protocol   d. Tell her that she should know better

21. You notice a coworker has been taking gauze every day from the supply cabinet. You should:

  a. Accuse him directly of stealing   b. Report it to a director   c. Tell another employee   d. Call the police

22. A parent requests a blanket for her child. When the nurse returns with the blanket, the parent says she has changed her mind. The nurse should:

  a. Express her disappointment   b. Leave the room without saying a word   c. Smile and tell the parent that it is fine   d. Calmly explain how the parent wasted precious time

23. Your director asks you to review some training materials that you have already seen. You should:

  a. Throw the materials away   b. Tell the director no   c. Review the materials as instructed   d. Ask an aide to review the materials and give you notes

24. You are really busy at work. Another coworker is crying because she cannot finish her duties for the day. You should:

  a. Help her complete her work   b. Tell her she needs to work harder   c. Stop what you are doing and counsel her   d. Encourage her to talk to a supervisor

25. You are off duty, and your supervisor sends you an email titled "EMERGENCY: PLEASE RESPOND ALL." You should:

  a. Ignore it because you are off duty   b. Respond as soon as possible   c. Delete it because it is ruining your work-life balance   d. Text your boss to privately complain

26. You have a scheduled break at 9:15 a.m. You need to call a family member, but it is only 8:45 a.m. You should:

  a. Take your break early to make the call   b. Ask someone to cover for you   c. Take the break at the scheduled time   d. Call quickly while on shift

27. You just remembered you forgot to sign some paperwork you recently filed. You should:

a. Continue the rest of your workday

b. Find the file and make sure it is signed

c. Ask a nurse's aide to sign on your behalf

d. Contact your supervisor immediately

28. You witnessed a coworker with whom you are close acquaintances break a rule, and your director interrogates you about her actions. What should you do?

a. Cover for her

b. Refuse to answer the questions

c. Report the truth

d. Say you will only speak to the director's supervisor

29. You forgot to clock out properly. How should you correct this error?

a. Clock out later next time

b. Ask a coworker to let your supervisor know what happened

c. Ask a coworker to clock out for you

d. Email your supervisor to apprise them of the mistake

30. A patient looks sad about his recent injury. How should you interact with him?

a. Tell him to cheer up

b. Ask him how you can help

c. Ask if he needs medication

d. Offer to get the practitioner

31. You see a family member pass a cigarette to a bedridden patient. The best thing to do is:

a. Act like you did not see anything

b. Take the cigarette from the patient

c. Ask the family member to leave

d. Politely explain hospital protocols

32. You are monitoring a young patient. You and the child are alone in the room when he slips out of bed and hits his head due to your negligence. You should respond by:

a. Helping the child back into bed and explaining that everything is okay

b. Restraining the child with straps so it does not happen again

c. Calling your attorney immediately before acting

d. Contacting your supervisor and documenting the events

33. A mother of a patient makes a derogatory comment about your appearance. What should you do?

a. Call security

b. Redirect the conversation

c. Get your supervisor

d. Tell her to leave the room

34. A patient forgot toothpaste. The nurse should:

a. Tell the patient to skip brushing her teeth

b. Tell her it is her problem

c. Provide toothpaste from stock

d. Call a family member

35. A patient makes some uncomfortable jokes about your body in your presence. The best thing to do is:

a. Refuse medical care to the patient

b. Call security immediately

c. Document the interaction and notify the supervisor

d. Get back at the patient by making another joke

36. You notice you are getting angry with a parent of a patient. You should:

a. Let them know your feelings

b. Take a moment to compose yourself, if possible

c. Get your supervisor

d. Tell them to leave you alone for a minute

37. A high-performing nurse always:

a. Follows directions with fidelity

b. Takes shortcuts when necessary

c. Speaks her mind assertively

d. Offers honest advice

38. A patient with a high fever keeps asking you to get him water even though you are busy. What should you do?

a. Focus on the other tasks you need to perform that day

b. Ignore the situation

c. Focus on helping the patient to the best of your ability

d. Show him how to get his own water

39. You witnessed a crime occur outside the office doors. The best approach is to:

a. Ignore it because it happened outside the office

b. Call the police to make a report

c. Chase the criminal off the premises

d. Tell the patients in the office to leave

40. A practitioner in your workplace is being sued for malpractice. A local news affiliate asks you for an official off-the-record comment. Your best response is to say:

a. "Malpractice happens. The media should stay out of our business."

b. "I am sorry. I would prefer not to comment on any legal matters."

c. "I am not surprised. I have worked with him for years."

d. "The patient is a liar. Plain and simple."

VOCATIONAL ADJUSTMENT INDEX

The following statements address certain personal or professional situations. Agreeing or disagreeing with the statements simply reveals how you are likely to think, feel, or act in certain circumstances. If you agree with the statement, select (A) in the corresponding row. If you disagree, select (D). Choose the answer that is most true for you and answer immediately. *Work rapidly.*

1.	People spend too much time focusing on their careers.	1.	(A)	(D)
2.	Most people are too competitive.	2.	(A)	(D)
3.	It is important to be a lifelong learner.	3.	(A)	(D)
4.	Collaboration is key to the success of any organization.	4.	(A)	(D)
5.	Most workplace evaluations are unfair.	5.	(A)	(D)
6.	Most older coworkers are out of touch.	6.	(A)	(D)
7.	People usually have the best intentions.	7.	(A)	(D)
8.	Working with others rather than alone is preferable.	8.	(A)	(D)
9.	It is important to take risks.	9.	(A)	(D)
10.	Efficiency is better than quality.	10.	(A)	(D)
11.	Kind hearts are for weak leaders.	11.	(A)	(D)
12.	A job is just a paycheck.	12.	(A)	(D)
13.	Conflict can be avoided through active listening.	13.	(A)	(D)
14.	Working with others is difficult.	14.	(A)	(D)
15.	Making rules is better than following rules.	15.	(A)	(D)
16.	Most coworkers are helpful.	16.	(A)	(D)
17.	Helping the elderly is rewarding.	17.	(A)	(D)
18.	Multitasking is difficult in collaborative settings.	18.	(A)	(D)
19.	Quiet environments are best for productivity.	19.	(A)	(D)
20.	Happiness is more important than financial stability.	20.	(A)	(D)
21.	You have to work for what you want.	21.	(A)	(D)
22.	Working with children is inspiring.	22.	(A)	(D)
23.	It is acceptable to be selfish in life.	23.	(A)	(D)
24.	Society is overly competitive.	24.	(A)	(D)
25.	Perfection is achievable.	25.	(A)	(D)
26.	An ideal job would be one without a strong workplace culture.	26.	(A)	(D)
27.	It is important to separate business and friendship in the workplace.	27.	(A)	(D)

28. It is difficult to make new friends.   28. Ⓐ Ⓓ

29. Success is more important than relationships.   29. Ⓐ Ⓓ

30. It is never acceptable to fail or lose.   30. Ⓐ Ⓓ

31. Social events are more exciting than alone time.   31. Ⓐ Ⓓ

32. Most supervisors are compassionate.   32. Ⓐ Ⓓ

33. It is more important to highlight someone's strengths than point out their weaknesses.   33. Ⓐ Ⓓ

34. Being radically candid is important.   34. Ⓐ Ⓓ

35. Unity is much more important than diversity.   35. Ⓐ Ⓓ

36. Most young people are clueless about the world.   36. Ⓐ Ⓓ

37. Everybody has the right to their own opinions.   37. Ⓐ Ⓓ

38. It is better to be vocal than to be submissive.   38. Ⓐ Ⓓ

39. It is better to be respected than feared.   39. Ⓐ Ⓓ

40. The best supervisors know how to delegate tasks to their workers.   40. Ⓐ Ⓓ

41. Seniority is more important than performance.   41. Ⓐ Ⓓ

42. The best workers are self-motivated.   42. Ⓐ Ⓓ

43. Discrimination does not really exist.   43. Ⓐ Ⓓ

44. It is important to make a list of daily tasks.   44. Ⓐ Ⓓ

45. An authority figure should never be contradicted.   45. Ⓐ Ⓓ

46. Some rules are meant to be broken.   46. Ⓐ Ⓓ

47. Employees should be fired if they make a mistake.   47. Ⓐ Ⓓ

48. People who complain are weak.   48. Ⓐ Ⓓ

49. Customers are normally difficult to work with.   49. Ⓐ Ⓓ

50. All leaders should be charismatic.   50. Ⓐ Ⓓ

51. Stress is hard to handle in the workplace.   51. Ⓐ Ⓓ

52. Teamwork is key to organizational success.   52. Ⓐ Ⓓ

53. There is one right path in life and many wrong paths.   53. Ⓐ Ⓓ

54. Money is the root of all evil.   54. Ⓐ Ⓓ

55. All people should be treated with dignity.   55. Ⓐ Ⓓ

56. Friendships with colleagues should be avoided.   56. Ⓐ Ⓓ

57. It feels good to be the center of attention.   57. Ⓐ Ⓓ

58. Most tasks at work are dehumanizing.   58. Ⓐ Ⓓ

59. Employee values should align in the workplace.   59. Ⓐ Ⓓ

60.	Most jobs consume too much time.	60.	(A)	(D)
61.	More elderly people need to retire earlier in life.	61.	(A)	(D)
62.	Disagreement is uncomfortable.	62.	(A)	(D)
63.	Sacrifice is important for team success.	63.	(A)	(D)
64.	Most police officers and security guards are uptight.	64.	(A)	(D)
65.	An ideal supervisor would be one who is direct and honest.	65.	(A)	(D)
66.	An ideal supervisor would be one who focuses on the details.	66.	(A)	(D)
67.	Most people foolishly just follow the rules.	67.	(A)	(D)
68.	Customer service is an important part of any job.	68.	(A)	(D)
69.	Cheating on an exam is never acceptable.	69.	(A)	(D)
70.	Many young people have all the best intentions.	70.	(A)	(D)
71.	The most stimulating environments are calm.	71.	(A)	(D)
72.	Large events are intimidating.	72.	(A)	(D)
73.	Sometimes it is necessary to take an unsanctioned break at work.	73.	(A)	(D)
74.	It is easy to reinvent yourself in new environments.	74.	(A)	(D)
75.	Conversation with strangers is quite easy.	75.	(A)	(D)
76.	Self-created goals are better than those created by others.	76.	(A)	(D)
77.	Flexibility is more important than structure.	77.	(A)	(D)
78.	Isolated work at a computer is better than collaborative work at a conference table.	78.	(A)	(D)
79.	Teachers often cater too much to student needs.	79.	(A)	(D)
80.	Variety is necessary for happiness.	80.	(A)	(D)
81.	Too many people are looking for a handout in this world.	81.	(A)	(D)
82.	People who have trouble choosing a career cannot be trusted as employees.	82.	(A)	(D)
83.	People who question norms are more likely to succeed in the workforce.	83.	(A)	(D)
84.	Every employee must always be on time, no matter the circumstance.	84.	(A)	(D)
85.	Every person deserves access to high-quality medical care.	85.	(A)	(D)
86.	It is unfair to break a promise to a colleague.	86.	(A)	(D)
87.	It is okay to give up when overwhelmed.	87.	(A)	(D)
88.	It is better to lie than hurt someone's feelings.	88.	(A)	(D)
89.	Silence is a sign of insecurity.	89.	(A)	(D)
90.	A series of smaller projects is preferable to one large project.	90.	(A)	(D)

Answer Key

Academic Aptitude: Verbal Skills

1. c.

Calm means "at ease or peaceful," and the other four words describe the feeling of being upset.

2. e.

Energetic means "wide awake or perky," and the other four words describe the need for rest.

3. d.

Certainty means "without a doubt," and the other four words describe issues or situations that need to be solved.

4. b.

Ordinary means "common or regular," and the other four words mean something strange or extraordinary.

5. c.

Thrive means "to grow in a positive way," and the other four words describe the inability to grow or the absence of growth.

6. b.

Thoughtless means "inconsiderate"; the other four words describe someone considerate and caring.

7. c.

Lacking means "missing or incomplete," and the other four words describe something that is complete or has all its parts.

8. c.

Bandage means "a covering for an injury," and the other four words are types of injuries.

9. a.

Lively means "upbeat or energetic," and the other four words refer to something lacking in positive energy.

10. d.

Long means "lengthy"; the other four words refer to something short or abrupt.

11. e.

Obvious means "understandable or apparent," and the other four words refer to something unknown, mysterious, or puzzling.

12. b.

Upbeat means "having a positive attitude," and the other four words refer to having a negative emotional state.

13. e.

Indifference means "disinterested"; the other four words refer to having an affection or liking for something.

14. e.

Rude means "showing a lack of manners or consideration," and the other four words refer to being friendly or agreeable.

15. d.

Divide means to "separate or disconnect," and the other four words refer to joining things together.

16. c.

Create means "to make something," and the other four words refer to destroying something.

17. b.

Drip means "trickle or drop," and the other four words refer to a heavy flow—usually of water or blood.

18. c.

Conflict means "a competition or lack of agreement," and the other four words describe a state of peace or harmony.

19. a.

Limited means "having defined boundaries," and the other four words refer to something that is never-ending.

20. d.

Disapprove means "condemn"; the other four words refer to forgiveness or approval.

21. b.

Humility means "modesty"; the other four words refer to being conceited.

22. e.

Perfect means "flawless"; the other four words refer to something flawed or defective.

23. d.

Conceited means "snobbish or arrogant," and the other four words refer to modesty and humbleness.

24. d.

Crude means "vulgar or rude," and the other four words refer to being well mannered.

25. e.

Serious means "thoughtful and sober," and the other four words refer to something ridiculous.

Academic Aptitude: Arithmetic

26. d.

Line up the decimals and add.

1.73

+ 2.17

3.90

27. a.

$24.17 + $32.87 = $57.04

$80.00 − $57.04 = **$22.96**

28. b.

Find the highest possible multiple of 4 that is less than or equal to 397, and then subtract to find the remainder.

99 × 4 = 396

397 − 396 = **1**

29. c.

If each student receives 2 notebooks, the teacher will need 16 × 2 = 32 notebooks. After handing out the notebooks, she will have 50 − 32 = **18 notebooks left**.

30. a.

Add the number of cupcakes he will give to his friend and to his coworkers, then subtract that value from 48.

# of cupcakes for his friend:

$\frac{1}{2} \times 48 = 24$

# of cupcakes for his coworkers:

$\frac{1}{3} \times 48 = 16$

48 − (24 + 16) = **8**

31. c.

Round each value and add.

129,113 ≈ 129,000

34,602 ≈ 35,000

129,000 + 35,000 = **164,000**

32. b.

There are 15 minutes between 7:45 a.m. and 8:00 a.m. and 20 minutes between 8:00 a.m. and 8:20 a.m.

15 minutes + 20 minutes = **35 minutes**

33. c.

23 ÷ 4 = 5.75 pizzas

Round up to **6 pizzas**.

34. e.

Use the formula for finding percentages. Express the percentage as a decimal.

part = whole × percentage = **1560 × 0.15**

35. b.

Multiply the cost per pound by the number of pounds purchased to find the cost of each fruit.

apples: 2(1.89) = 3.78

oranges: 1.5(2.19) = 3.285

3.78 + 3.285 = 7.065 = **$7.07**

36. c.

Divide 1.3208 by 5.2.

$$
\begin{array}{r}
.254 \\
52\overline{)13.208} \\
\underline{104} \\
280 \\
\underline{260} \\
208 \\
\underline{208} \\
0
\end{array}
$$

37. b.

Align the decimals and add/subtract from left to right.

$17.38 - 19.26 + 14.2$

$= (-1.88) + 14.2 = \textbf{12.32}$

38. e.

Write a proportion and then solve for x.

$\frac{40}{45} = \frac{265}{x}$

$40x = 11,925$

$x = 298.125 \approx \textbf{298}$

39. b.

$\frac{1}{4} = \frac{x}{20}$

$4x = 20$

$x = \textbf{5}$

40. c.

$\frac{25}{2} = \frac{x}{8}$

$2x = 200$

$x = \textbf{100}$

41. a.

$0.8 + 0.49 + 0.89 = 2.18$

$2.5 - 2.18 = \textbf{0.32}$

42. c.

Line up the decimals and subtract.

$$
\begin{array}{r}
4.50 \\
- 1.67 \\
\hline
\textbf{2.83}
\end{array}
$$

43. a.

$\$285.48 \div 6 = \textbf{\$47.58}$

44. c.

Line up the decimals and subtract.

$$
\begin{array}{r}
119.70 \\
- 1.05 \\
\hline
\textbf{118.65}
\end{array}
$$

45. c.

$\$25.44 \div 3.2 = \textbf{\$7.95}$

46. a.

$6.3 \div 18 = \textbf{0.35 lb}$

47. d.

48 cents = $0.48

$\$1.68 \div \$0.48 = \textbf{3.5}$

48. c.

$127 - 150 = 127 + (-150) = \textbf{-23}$

49. a.

The average of five numbers is the sum of the numbers divided by 5. Multiply the average by 5 to find the sum; subtract to find the fifth number.

$\frac{sum}{5} = 16$

$sum = 16 \times 5 = 80$

$80 - 68 = \textbf{12}$

50. a.

$\frac{4}{50} = \frac{x}{175}$

$50x = 700$

$x = \textbf{14 mL}$

Academic Aptitude: Nonverbal Skills

51.	b.	64.	a.
52.	a.	65.	a.
53.	e.	66.	b.
54.	a.	67.	c.
55.	c.	68.	d.
56.	e.	69.	a.
57.	d.	70.	b.
58.	c.	71.	d.
59.	c.	72.	b.
60.	a.	73.	c.
61.	a.	74.	e.
62.	c.	75.	c.
63.	e.		

Spelling

1.	a. muscle	24.	a. symptom
2.	c. hormone	25.	c. eliminate
3.	b. seizure	26.	b. adhere
4.	c. facilities	27.	b. enable
5.	a. decrease	28.	b. various
6.	a. transfusion	29.	c. secretion
7.	b. anatomy	30.	c. trauma
8.	b. diagnosis	31.	c. excessive
9.	c. equipment	32.	a. bacteria
10.	a. stomach	33.	c. fungus
11.	b. arthritis	34.	b. monitor
12.	b. ovary	35.	c. abrasion
13.	a. surgical	36.	c. multiple
14.	c. allergy	37.	a. tremor
15.	a. inflammation	38.	c. involvement
16.	c. poison	39.	c. respiratory
17.	a. atrophy	40.	b. cranial
18.	b. sterile	41.	c. disease
19.	a. cellular	42.	a. artery
20.	b. tissue	43.	b. vein
21.	b. artificial	44.	b. chronic
22.	c. immediate	45.	c. acute
23.	c. droplet		

General Science

1. a.

   Calcium is the most abundant mineral found in bones, as well as in the entire body.

2. d.

   A biome is a large ecological community that includes specific plants and animals; a desert is one example.

3. b.

   Venus's orbit is closest to Earth. Venus is the second planet from the sun, and Earth is the third planet from the sun.

4. e.

   Before a star collapses, the star burns brighter for a period of time and then fades from view. This is a supernova.

5. c.

   Tulips are plants, meaning they have chloroplasts to perform photosynthesis.

6. c.

   Isotopes are atoms of the same element with the same number of protons but different numbers of neutrons.

7. d.

   Tachycardia is an abnormally fast heart rate, and electrocardiograms show the electrical activity of the heart.

8. a.

   Each codon contains three nucleotides.

9. c.

   Electrons are negatively charged particles in an atom; electrons orbit the nucleus.

10. a.

    Tension is the force that results from objects being pulled or hung.

11. b.

    Mushrooms are fungi. Fungi break down organic material left by dead animals and plants, making them decomposers.

12. d.

    The metabolic rate of crustaceans, such as lobsters, is too low to regulate their temperature. Crustaceans use behavioral techniques, such as moving to shallow water, to maintain body temperature.

13. d.

    The tibia is a lower leg bone.

14. e.

    The digestive enzymes produced by the pancreas pass into the small intestine.

15. a.

    When water changes form, it does not change the chemical composition of the substance. Once water becomes ice, the ice can easily turn back into water.

16. c.

    Coal is nonrenewable because once coal is burned, it cannot be quickly replaced.

17. b.

    The lithosphere is the top layer of the earth's surface.

18. c.

    The skeletal muscles and the bone are attached by the tendons.

19. a.

    The esophagus is the muscular passageway through which food travels on its way from the mouth to the stomach.

20. b.

    Earth takes approximately twenty-four hours to rotate on its axis.

21. d.

    Photosynthesis is the process by which plants convert the energy of the sun into stored chemical energy (glucose).

22. d.

    Combustion is defined as a reaction in which a hydrocarbon reacts with O_2 to produce CO_2 and H_2O.

23. e.

Nonliving things in an ecosystem, like air and water, are abiotic factors.

24. e.

Most fungi derive their energy by breaking down dead plant and animal matter.

25. e.

The mechanism of natural selection is rooted in the idea that there is variation in inherited traits among a population of organisms, resulting in differential reproduction.

26. b.

The tongue is the muscle that helps break apart food, mix it with saliva, and direct it toward the esophagus.

27. a.

When placed in water, strong acids immediately break apart into their constituent ions.

28. d.

The femur is the largest bone of the human body.

29. d.

Sunlight helps the skin produce vitamin D.

30. b.

The light reactions of photosynthesis occur in the chloroplast. Each chloroplast has stacks of membranes called thylakoids where enzymes convert light energy into chemical energy.

31. c.

Capillaries enable exchange of cellular waste, gases, and nutrients on the cellular level.

32. c.

The incus, stapes, and malleus are bones connected to the skull that play an important role in the sense of hearing.

33. c.

Adrenal glands sit on top of each kidney.

34. c.

An anemometer measures wind speed.

35. e.

$1\ ml = 1\ cm^3$

36. d.

Mature sperm are stored in the epididymis.

37. a.

Meninges are present only in the dorsal cavity that holds the spinal cord and brain.

38. a.

Organic compounds may contain phosphorous, nitrogen, or oxygen, but they *must* contain carbon.

39. e.

Nucleic acids (DNA and RNA) are composed of nucleotides. Each nucleotide is composed of a five-carbon sugar, a nitrogenous base, and a phosphate group.

40. d.

Uracil is found in RNA but not in DNA.

41. b.

Gametes (sperm and egg) have half the number of chromosomes contained in an organism's somatic cells.

42. c.

An ax is an example of a wedge.

43. a.

The valence shell of the noble gases (group 18) is full, so these gases do not need to add electrons.

44. e.

Through photosynthesis, leaves use the sun's energy to convert carbon dioxide into glucose.

45. d.

Deposition occurs when a gas becomes a solid.

46. a.

Acids have a pH between 0 and 7.

47. e.

A balance measures mass.

48. b.

Friction occurs when motion is impeded because one object is rubbing against another object.

49. a.

Igneous rocks form when liquid rock cools and solidifies.

50. c.

Sound waves are longitudinal waves because the vibrations travel in the same direction as the energy.

51. c.

Nitrogen makes up 78 percent of Earth's atmosphere.

52. c.

All atoms of the same element contain the same number of protons.

53. e.

Hydrogen is the most common element in the universe.

54. d.

Tornadoes occur when warm air masses collide with cold air masses over land.

55. a.

Baking soda (sodium bicarbonate) is a base, which will neutralize an acid.

56. b.

Gravity is a force that attracts objects to the center of the earth or toward other objects having mass.

57. e.

Potential energy is energy that is stored and waiting to work.

58. c.

A T-shirt is translucent; it lets some light pass through.

59. c.

A marble is an example of an electrical insulator—it stops the transfer of electrical energy. The other choices are all electrical conductors.

60. a.

Stratus clouds are often gray.

Judgment and Comprehension

1. b.

Rationale: You are the only one responsible for documenting your patient care; delegating this task is not appropriate. Continuing to try is important, but discussing it with the supervisor may help you find solutions to the problem.

2. c.

Rationale: Speaking to the nurse privately and directly is the best way to address the issue. Continuing to help will perpetuate the problem, and calling a coworker lazy does not promote a healthy work environment. The nurse should discuss this with the supervisor before calling HR.

3. a.

Rationale: It is not appropriate to ask a coworker to cover this employee's duties while he takes an unapproved and unscheduled break from work. Politely refusing is sufficient and avoids insult, which the other responses do not.

4. d.

Rationale: Addressing the parent directly about the child's behavior is the most appropriate action. The other responses are judgmental and do not demonstrate therapeutic communication.

5. c.

Rationale: Reassuring the patient and offering assistance is the best response. Dismissing or ridiculing his feelings is unprofessional and demonstrates a lack of compassion for patient concerns. The other options are not therapeutic.

6. a.

Rationale: It is a violation of HIPPA and would be unprofessional to allow this woman to see the patient. The police cannot intervene, and the nurse should not make the patient deal with this woman.

7. b.

Rationale: Reviewing policies and contacting the supervisor are the most accurate and direct ways to handle this situation. You are responsible for taking appropriate action when ill and should not ask a coworker to help. Taking time off without notification can lead to termination, and going in to work while sick poses an infection control concern.

8. a.

Rationale: You should consult the practitioner if the patient appears to be reacting in an unexpected way to medication. Telling the patient he is having an allergic or adverse reaction will increase his anxiety. The patient's concerns should not be dismissed without offering help.

9. c.

Rationale: Asking for help is the best approach in this situation. A supervisor likely has more flexibility and ability to spend time assisting you. It is unsafe to attempt a procedure if you do not feel you can carry it out correctly, and you should not avoid it just because you do not remember how to do it.

10. c.

Rationale: If a nurse is not working, it is important to address the situation with the lead nurse or a supervisor, as it could present a patient safety issue. Calling a coworker lazy does not support a healthy work environment, nor does taking a photo of her without consent. Security has no influence over this situation.

11. c.

Rationale: The patient should not be given anyone's personal email address, but he should be given the information needed to lodge a complaint or comment if he requests it. Providing a fake email or one's own email is unprofessional, as is telling the patient he is ridiculous.

12. b.

Rationale: It is the nurse's responsibility to be honest and have integrity in patient care. Leaving the scene would constitute abandonment of the patient, and calling a lawyer is unnecessary. Asking a visitor for help would violate the patient's privacy. The best course of action is to call the supervising nurse.

13. b.

Rationale: Providing reassurance to the patient is the best approach in this situation. The other responses are not therapeutic and may make the patient feel worse.

14. b.

Rationale: Every patient, despite their condition, should be treated the same way. Making exceptions to rules can be detrimental to the patient care plan. Counsel through prayer is not appropriate for a nurse, and speaking directly about the tumor would only be appropriate if the child spoke about it first.

15. b.

Rationale: You should determine the nature and characteristics of the pain to best guide the patient to the correct level of care. Only the provider can make a diagnosis, and discussing possible illnesses is inappropriate and serves no purpose in this situation. Distracting the patient from the pain is appropriate after assessing the pain.

16. c.

Rationale: Explain the organizational policy to this family member. Make it clear that no home medications or outside medications are to be administered, and doing so may harm the patient. It is not necessary to remove the family member, and her credentials are not pertinent to this situation. Using the word "stupid" is never appropriate or professional.

17. d.

Rationale: A foundational understanding of the profession is a priority for success; customer service is important, but it cannot be effectively provided without that understanding. Flexibility and experimentation are not appropriate choices, as all actions and interventions must be supported by evidence-based practice.

18. b.

Rationale: Discussing the matter privately may allow for some consideration to be made on your behalf. Asking the supervisor for help or delegating the tasks may be necessary. If you feel certain you will fail, you should be proactive in getting help. Telling your supervisor he is expecting too much might be viewed as insubordination. Quitting is an option, but not necessarily the best one.

19. a.

Rationale: Providing a step-by-step explanation will help the patient understand the process and know what to expect. The other options are not inappropriate, but they do not help the patient to feel safe and comfortable. Not speaking to the patient would likely seem awkward and could present a safety issue.

20. c.

Rationale: Reminding the supervisor of the protocol is the best way to address this situation. It should be done objectively, professionally, and respectfully. Suggesting she should know better is unprofessional, and contacting a legal representative is not necessary. Quitting on the spot is an option but is likely not the best course of action.

21. b.

Rationale: The staff is responsible for appropriate use of resources. It is not ethical to take supplies for personal use, and this should be reported to a director if witnessed. It is not appropriate to call the police. Speaking to another employee would be unprofessional, and accusing the coworker directly may lead to a poor outcome.

22. c.

Rationale: It would not serve any constructive purpose to express disappointment, explain about time wasted, or be rude by leaving without speaking. The nurse can leave the blanket for later use and provide reassurance to the patient and the family.

23. c.

Rationale: If a director or supervisor instructs a nurse to perform an action, they should do so. Throwing the materials away or saying no is insubordination. It would be inappropriate to delegate such a task to an aide.

24. d.

Rationale: A supervisor has the authority to assist with redistribution or delegation of work. It is not within your scope as a peer to counsel the nurse, and it may be difficult to help if you are already busy. Suggesting she work harder does not help solve the problem.

25. b.

Rationale: The nurse should always respond to emergency communications as soon as possible. As a public servant, you should be ready to perform any duty related to that role. You should not delete or ignore the email, nor should you complain via text message.

26. c.

Rationale: The nurse should not make phone calls during work time. It is not appropriate to change a scheduled break time or ask a coworker to cover for you. If there is an emergency, the nurse should consult a supervisor.

27. b.

Rationale: As a nurse, you are obligated to perform work to the best of your ability, completely and accurately. There is no need to contact the supervisor if you can correct the situation yourself, and you should not ask anyone to sign on your behalf.

28. c.

Rationale: The nurse is obligated to report the truth in an objective manner. It is generally appropriate to honor the chain of command in leadership, and therefore reporting to the director is suggested. Refusing to answer the question can compromise patient safety issues, as can as covering for the coworker.

29. d.

Rationale: The nurse should take responsibility for the action and notify the supervisor as soon as possible. Asking a coworker to do it is not appropriate. The nurse should make every effort to clock out at the right time after each period of work.

30. b.

Rationale: If a patient appears sad, it is appropriate to start a discussion about how you can help. Allow him to express his feelings and use good listening skills. It is not necessary to get the practitioner before discussing the concern with the patient, and offering medication is not appropriate. Suggesting that the patient cheer up may alienate him.

31. d.

Rationale: Politely explain hospital protocols to the family member, then remove the lit cigarette from the room. The family member should be asked to leave if they continue to defy the policy. The nurse should not ignore the action.

32. d.

Rationale: A patient fall from a bed is a serious safety issue, and a possible head injury should be documented. The nurse should notify the supervisor, but there is no need to call an attorney. It is unethical and poor practice to restrain the child. It is appropriate to help the child into bed and reassure him, but documentation and notification are essential.

33. b.

Rationale: Redirecting the conversation should divert the woman from making further comments. While inappropriate, such comments do not constitute harassment or abuse, but if the situation escalates, you should contact your supervisor. It is not appropriate to ask the woman to leave the room, and calling security would be an overreaction.

34. c.

Rationale: Basic hygiene items should be provided to patients so they can maintain personal care. Asking the patient to skip performing hygiene is not appropriate, and calling a family member is not the best course of action. It is never appropriate to tell a patient that something is their problem or to dismiss their needs.

35. c.

Rationale: The nurse should document the interaction objectively and notify the supervisor of the behavior. While you should not tolerate the behavior, you should not retaliate. Calling security is not appropriate in this situation, and it is unethical to refuse medical care to a patient for making jokes.

36. b.

Rationale: Taking a moment to compose yourself is the best approach. Getting angry may be a sign that you are too emotionally invested in the situation. The nurse should not express anger to patients. A secondary option is to speak to your supervisor for advice, but they should not be necessary to finding composure and continuing patient care.

37. a.

Rationale: Fidelity is an ethical principle that requires nurses to be faithful to their profession and all related professional constructs. Taking shortcuts violates that faith. Speaking one's mind is not a violation of fidelity, but it should be done at the right place and time, and with the right intent. Offering advice is generally not in the scope of the nurse, but advocacy is.

38. c.

Rationale: The patient should always be the priority. Most tasks not directly related to patient care are not as important as addressing patient needs. Ignoring patients is never appropriate, and showing patients how to get their own water would require them to leave their room, which may compromise safety as well as infection control.

39. b.

Rationale: If the crime does not occur in the workplace, it is best to phone the police to report it. While waiting for the police to arrive, it is appropriate to notify staff of the crime in case safety measures need to be taken. Chasing the criminal or asking the patients to leave may put people in danger, and ignoring the crime would not be ethical.

40. b.

Rationale: The best response is to make no comment. Most health care facilities have a policy that governs staff members' boundaries when speaking to the media. Any other response would not be appropriate and would likely result in disciplinary action.

Vocational Adjustment Index

There is no "right" answer to the questions on the Vocational Adjustment Index. Every school will interpret your score differently, so just focus on answering the questions quickly and honestly.

Follow the link below to take your second PSB APNE practice test:

www.ascenciatestprep.com/psb-apne-online-resources

Made in the USA
Middletown, DE
15 June 2019